VICTORY
OVER ADHD

Deborah Merlin

HEALTHY LIVING PUBLICATIONS
Summertown, Tennessee

Library of Congress Cataloging-in-Publication Data

Merlin, Deborah.
   Victory over ADHD / by Deborah Merlin.
      p. cm.
   Includes bibliographical references.
  ISBN 978-1-57067-234-7
1. Attention-deficit hyperactivity disorder—Alternative treatment. I.
Title.
   RJ506.H9M48 2009
   618.92'8589—dc22

                           2009015383

Book Publishing Co. is a member of Green Press Initiative. We chose to print this title on paper with postconsumer recycled content, processed without chlorine, which saved the following natural resources:

48 trees

2,247 pounds of solid waste

17,456 gallons of wastewater

4,226 pounds of greenhouse gases

33 million BTU of total energy

green press INITIATIVE

BOOK PUBLISHING COMPANY

For more information, visit www.greenpressinitiative.org.

Paper calculations from Environmental Defense Paper Calculator, www.edf.org/papercalculator.

Printed in Canada

Healthy Living Publications
a division of Book Publishing Company
P.O. Box 99
Summertown, TN 38483
888-260-8458
www.bookpubco.com

ISBN 978-1-57067-234-7

17 16 15 14 13 12 11 10 09   1 2 3 4 5 6 7 8 9

DEDICATION

In memory of Judith Bluestone,

educator, intuitive healer,

founder of The HANDLE Institute,

and internationally renowned authority

on neurodevelopmental disorders.

Contents

An epidemic of problems affects our children in this twenty-first century. We have the usual problems of drug abuse, delinquency, and the uncertainty of the future, but in addition to these important issues, we are faced with an unprecedented rise in autism and ADHD. These complex conditions often overwhelm the average person's ability to understand and therefore seek effective treatment.

As a physician, I have various treatment options for ADHD, autism, and other psychiatric problems in children. The conventional medical treatments consist mainly of various prescription medications. Although effective in some cases, prescription drugs also have many negative side effects that limit their use. However, there are numerous alternative treatments that don't use drugs or have significant side effects. These alternative approaches may include nutrition improvement, vitamin supplementation, elimination of foods known to cause allergies, heavy metal detoxification, balancing of neurotransmitters by amino acids, acupuncture, and herbs to help address root causes and then strengthen, build, and repair weakened bodily systems. The elimination of *Candida* and parasites from the bowel is often included in alternative treatments yet ignored by conventional medicine.

I am often shocked by how quickly a child is placed on a medication—such as Ritalin—without the investigation of safe, natural alternatives. The need for the education of parents and their children about alternative medicine and lifestyle choices is the reason why I'm enthusiastically writing this foreword for Deborah's story.

Deborah Merlin—mother of two premature infants—had the courage and the tenacity to do everything possible to ensure that her children grew up to be normal, healthy adults. As you will discover, the task was not easy. Westley and Erik, whom I have examined at the clinic, are now wonderful young adults. Their story is an immensely interesting journey through many doctors and philosophies. Deborah had been given conflicting diagnoses, often with opposing suggested treatments, yet she remained steadfast in seeking what made sense to her as a mother. Often the "nonprofessional" mother is more correct than the experts.

This book fills an important need—it's an idea whose time has come. For all the mothers and fathers who are confused and searching, this book will bring clarity. I know this book will open a whole new possibility for the many parents and children who read it.

David R. Allen, MD
www.drallmd.org

Preface

The Fly's Lesson

When my kids were young, I was constantly sick with bronchitis, ear infections, vertigo, vitiligo, Hashimoto's thyroiditis, chronic fatigue, and headaches. My children had chronic ear and sinus infections, allergies, and ADHD. We all took antibiotics more often than not.

Once my children went off to school, I would go straight back to bed and rest until they came home. One warm morning as I lay in bed, a fly dashed into my room. Relentlessly, he banged against the window screen, trying to escape.

I identified with that fly; I was in a trap of my own. No matter how many times we visited the doctor or took antibiotics, we didn't get well. In fact, we got sicker.

If only the fly had flown out through the living room into the kitchen, he could have fled through the doggy door. It was probably the way he got inside in the first place. That was when I had my "Aha!" moment.

Whatever I did wasn't working, and I needed a new and different approach to heal myself and my children. This brought me to the first step on the path to alternative medicine.

Deborah Merlin

Acknowledgments

I wish to express special gratitude to all the health care professionals and experts who contributed their writing and articles to this book: Judith Bluestone, James P. Blumenthal, Rashid A. Buttar, Pat Farrell, Stuart H. Garber, Dan O. Harper, Janet Starr Hull, Jack Johnstone, Kathleen Lewis, Debbie Lindgren, Marlene McKee, Tricia Ann Ochoa, Emily Roberts, Barbara Schwartz, Jane Sheppard, and Lesa Werner. Without their invaluable help and expertise this book would not have been possible.

I am forever indebted to my dear friend the late Pamela Healey, who connected me to many of the people instrumental in writing the chapters of this book.

My deepest appreciation goes to my children, Erik and Westley, for teaching me about motherhood on the deepest level, and to my husband, Chris, for having the wisdom to say no to Ritalin and for supporting my mission to write this book.

Many thanks to my mother, Joan McCausland; my father, Gordon Reinauer; my sister Kathryn Payette; my brother David Reinauer; my brother-in-law Mark Merlin; and my sister-in-law Sally Merlin.

I am eternally grateful to David R. Allen for thinking outside the box and for healing my children by addressing causes, not just symptoms. Thank you also for writing the foreword to this book.

I am especially grateful to my friends Glenna Citron, Sigrid Macdonald, and Katherine Redwine for reading the manuscript, offering their suggestions, and providing unconditional love and support. Thank you to all the enlightened women in our wisdom circle. Special gratitude to Toni Galardi for her support and inspiration.

Much appreciation goes to Jesse Merlin and Kay Neth for their invaluable help editing, and to Larry Cook, my former collaborator, for his guidance and support.

SECTION

The Journey

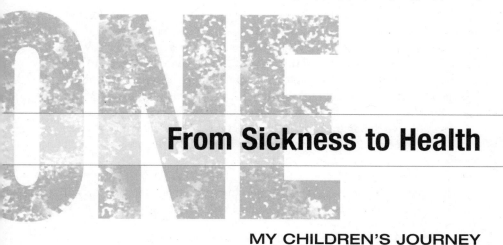

CHAPTER 1

From Sickness to Health

MY CHILDREN'S JOURNEY

I f you've picked up this book, you're probably curious about natural living. You want to make wise choices for you and your family. Maybe you'd like to know more about alternative medicine. Perhaps you have a child with an attention disorder, behavioral difficulties, or neurological problems—and you want solutions.

You've come to the right place.

I spent a great deal of time, energy, and money looking for solutions for my children—two young boys who were diagnosed with attention disorders by the time they were three years old. It would take me seven years of searching to find what my children really needed to address their problems. And the solutions had nothing to do with Ritalin or other conventional medical approaches. The answers lay in improving my children's diet, discovering and addressing nutritional deficiencies, and turning to other natural approaches. Along the way, I discovered the lifestyle choices that I had to make to live optimally, healthfully, and happily.

Once I figured out what my boys needed to thrive, the results were dramatic. Exploring natural remedies during our seven-year journey toward health and well-being was well worth my time. But you can begin the healing process faster than I did by using the information and resources on pages 179–181 of this book.

Love, Marriage, and Pregnancy

I was thirty-three years old and single, working as an insurance inspector and living in an apartment in Santa Monica, California. I drove a red MR2 Toyota sports car and worked out at the gym every day. I was having a good time, though my life lacked substance.

I met Chris at the gym one Sunday morning in an aerobics class. We were married thirty-two days after our first date. We were madly in love, and I wanted to get pregnant right away. He wanted to wait two years, so we compromised and decided to start trying to get pregnant in a year. Chris understandably wanted to spend some time alone with me, but I was concerned about my biological clock.

At an ob-gyn appointment, I told my doctor that I planned to start trying to conceive in three months, which would have been June 1. It would take a while, my doctor warned, because I was thirty-four years old.

I conceived on June 4.

Unfortunately, conceiving was the only easy thing about my pregnancy.

When I was about six weeks pregnant, I did a light workout at the gym. I went home, took a shower and started to make breakfast. Suddenly, I felt my legs become damp. I looked under my bathrobe—blood was streaming down my legs. In a panic I called my doctor. He told me there was a 50 percent chance that I would miscarry—but the fact that I wasn't experiencing cramps was a good sign.

The next morning, Chris and I went to see the doctor, who, to our relief, determined that I was still pregnant. We scheduled an ultrasound for the following Friday.

That night I dreamed I was back where I grew up on the East Coast, wearing a blue maternity dress, telling my family that I was expecting twins. The following morning I told my husband about the dream. He quickly interrupted me. Twins, Chris groaned, would be his worst nightmare—the extra responsibility, the expense.

The following Friday I went to have the ultrasound while Chris was at work.

The monitor showed two hearts beating.

Twins.

After the ultrasound, my doctor warned me that I would probably have another bleeding episode at three months. A twin pregnancy would be a totally different ballgame, he noted. I would have to stop working at six months and spend the duration of the pregnancy in bed.

I felt a little scared—and excited. But how would Chris react to the news?

When he arrived home, I took him into the bedroom and sat him down. Chris asked me how the ultrasound went. I told him I was still pregnant. And we were going to have twins.

Chris was speechless. He got his voice back twenty-four hours later. Before long he was bragging to everyone that we were expecting two babies, not just one.

As my doctor had predicted, I had a bleeding episode at three months. He also told me that twins tend to be born early, and if I went into premature labor, medicines could stop the contractions, provided I received immediate medical attention.

The second bleeding stopped, and I was doing well. My doctor had nixed exercise. But I continued to work full time, even as I was becoming larger than I ever would have imagined. I looked ridiculous driving a little red sports car.

My last day of work was the day before Thanksgiving. The next day, I didn't feel well. Nonetheless, we drove to my mother-in-law's house for dinner in our brand new station wagon. I ate modestly, but shortly after dinner I felt nauseated. My mother-in-law told me I looked gray. I wanted to go home—to throw up in private. I was sure we could make it to our house in time; we lived just a mile away. But the ride felt like an eternity.

As we pulled into the driveway, I threw up all over the inside of our new car. I stumbled from the car and then threw up on the lawn. Chris took out the garden hose and washed down the yard.

By morning my vomiting had finally stopped. I was exhausted. I felt some cramping and was experiencing flulike symptoms. By evening the cramping was more intense, so I called my doctor, who told me to go the emergency room immediately.

By the time I arrived at the hospital, my contractions were four minutes apart and my cervix had dilated a centimeter. I was only twenty-seven weeks pregnant—most pregnancies last about thirty-six weeks.

The nurse set up an IV drip with terbutaline to stop the contractions. The contractions slowed, but when my doctor examined me the next morning, his expression showed panic. My cervix was 90 percent effaced. (Although effacement, the thinning of the cervix, is a normal part of the body's preparation for birth, 100 percent effacement should not happen until the last month of pregnancy, shortly before the child is born.) I would have to spend the duration of the pregnancy in the hospital, in bed, with my lower body elevated to prevent pressure on my cervix.

My husband was working twelve hours a day. He had a young son, who was living with us and who needed his father, too. I don't know how Chris did it all. He would rush home from work to feed his son, then come to the hospital and hold my hand every night. He took care of everything. It was a special time for us, and we became even closer.

The terbutaline made my heart race and gave me severe heartburn. After several days, my contractions stopped, and the nurse took me off the IV. I started taking the terbutaline orally, and I was moved out of intensive care. I could get up only to use the restroom. I spent the next several days in bed, my lower body elevated.

I always looked forward to my next meal, and the hospital food was actually quite good. By the twenty-ninth week, I looked like a beached whale. I was enormous. But it didn't matter. Every day I kept the pregnancy going increased the chances of my twins' survival.

After spending eighteen days in bed, my mood darkened. I grew irritable. The heartburn would not let up, and I was developing painful bedsores. I missed being single. I feared that the pregnancy was a mistake. I decided my biological clock had played a mean trick on me, making me believe I wanted to be a mother. I was clueless about motherhood. I had never even changed a diaper.

The next night the contractions returned. I called the nurse. It was evident that I was in labor again. She set up an IV drip. The terbutaline was no longer working, and the nurse switched the medicine to magnesium. But by the following night the contractions had grown more intense.

Chris spent the night at the hospital by my side. He stayed awake all night and felt every contraction with me.

The Birth

It was Friday morning, and I had been in labor thirty-two hours. My doctor arrived shortly after 8:00 a.m. He examined me and discovered that I was four and a half centimeters dilated and one of the twins was breeched—in other words, the hind end of his body would emerge first. The doctor said he would have to perform an emergency Cesarean section, and he left the room to prepare for surgery.

Chris came to my bed and held me as we both wept. I was only thirty weeks pregnant.

I was wheeled into surgery around 9:00 a.m. The anesthesiologist prepared me for a spinal block. My doctor and his colleague came in to deliver the twins. Two more doctors came in from the neonatal intensive care unit (NICU); each of the four doctors had a nurse to assist him. Including my husband and me, twelve people were in the delivery room.

Everything seemed surreal, though the mood was relaxed. I felt no pain as the doctor made the incision. At 9:20 a.m., the first twin was delivered. My husband cried. He cut the umbilical cord. We named our firstborn Erik. He weighed three pounds and two ounces, a good weight, I was told, considering how premature he was. Doctors use the Apgar scale to determine a newborn's level of health. Ten is the highest score. At birth, Erik's score was eight; five minutes later he was upgraded to nine. Before the nurse took Erik to the NICU, she paused briefly so I could kiss him on the forehead.

Chris was full of emotion as the doctors struggled to deliver the second twin, who put up a good fight. The mood changed, and there was no time for my husband to cut the umbilical cord. The baby was dark blue and had to be rushed to the NICU. I didn't even get a glimpse of him. His Apgar score was four, though five minutes later it was upgraded to a nine. I was told he weighed three pounds and four ounces. We named him Westley.

I don't recall leaving the delivery room. I woke up, disoriented, in the recovery room. The doctor from the NICU paid me a visit. He told me the first twin was doing better than expected; however, Westley had challenges. His lungs were underdeveloped, resulting in hyaline membrane disease. The next forty-eight hours were critical. Both the boys were in incubators.

I felt fatigued and too ill to see my babies. After a bedridden three weeks, I'd developed pneumonia. Chris brought in a Polaroid picture of the boys for me. I never let that photo out of my sight.

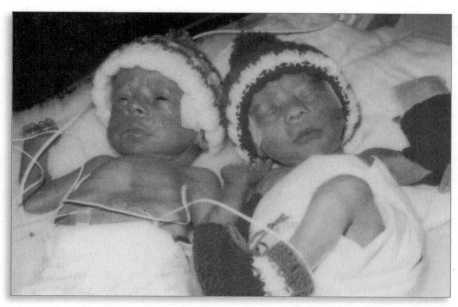

Westley and Erik in NICU. Notice Westley's sunken chest.

I was unable to visit the NICU until the third day. I held Erik first. He was tiny. He opened his eyes and looked right at me. I knew he couldn't actually see me, but my heart swelled with love.

The NICU was a busy and noisy place. I wanted to be alone to bond with my babies. I knew the nurses were observing me, and it made me feel uncomfortable. I gave Erik back to the nurse and walked to Westley's incubator. He was hooked up to a ventilator, with several wires attached to him. His underdeveloped lungs had caused his chest to appear concave. I watched him for a few minutes and returned to my room to cry. If only I could have carried the pregnancy a few more weeks. I felt like a failure.

The boys would have to stay in the NICU for several weeks so they could develop a sucking reflex to take in enough fluids and gain weight. It felt strange leaving the hospital without them. I visited them every day, as I had to pump milk from my breasts every three hours to supply them with nourishment. Fortunately, my milk supply was abundant.

When the boys were three weeks old, the doctor told us Westley had developed a staph infection and meningitis, and Erik had bleeding from his rectum. And there was more bad news: the doctor warned us that Erik might have necrotizing enterocolitis, a sometimes fatal disease that destroys all or part of a baby's bowel.

Both babies were started on antibiotics. The staff said someone would call us if the twins took a turn for the worse.

The phone rang at two o'clock in the morning. My heart raced. I thought the nurses were calling to say both boys had died. My husband answered the phone. It was his sister; she wanted us to know that my mother-in-law had been admitted to the hospital that night. Needless to say, we were concerned but relieved; still, I could not go back to sleep. The next day the boys were improving, and we learned that Erik didn't have narcotizing enterocolitis after all.

At seven weeks Erik was ready to go home. He weighed a whopping five pounds—he hadn't been due to be born for three more weeks. He cried every two hours to be fed. I was exhausted and could not imagine having another baby to take care of.

Westley had to remain on the ventilator for one month after his birth. Once he was removed from the ventilator, he was put on oxygen for the next two and a half months. I took Erik with me every day to visit Westley, who, at that point, was described by the hospital as having a "failure to thrive." He had difficulty sucking from his bottle. The nurses would heat my breast milk so I could feed him, and it took what seemed like forever to get any substantial amount of milk into him. Westley remained withdrawn, and I struggled to bond with him. I watched all the other preemies go home as he remained behind. I was tired of going to the NICU every day, yet I could not bring him home the way he was.

Going Home

After three and a half months, Westley no longer required oxygen; however, er, he was still a slow feeder. The doctors gave him steroid injections, and he slowly improved. At four months the doctors decided he was ready to go home. He weighed seven and a half pounds and could take in only sixteen ounces of milk a day. A doctor warned us that he would either sink or swim.

Westley was sent home wearing an apnea monitor, a device for observing heart function. At home, he took in less and less milk as the days passed. He wouldn't wake up to be fed and refused to take a bottle when I woke him. By the eighth day, he was taking in just eight ounces of milk every twenty-four hours. I took him to the pediatrician, and Westley was readmitted to the hospital.

Westley had an enlarged liver—hepatomegaly—because of fluid retention, and he was given a diuretic called Lasix (generically known as furosemide) as well as other diuretic medicines. He returned from the hospital after a few days, still on diuretics. He remained withdrawn, made little eye contact, and cried when I held him. It was evident that we would need help with Westley. We were at a loss, and the social worker at the hospital suggested that we hire a nurse to feed him at night.

The nurse arrived regularly at 8:00 p.m. and inserted a gavage feeding tube into Westley's nose, passed it down into his stomach, and fed him. It wasn't easy. Westley screamed and arched his back, and sometimes made it impossible to insert the tube. Before long he had to be readmitted to the hospital for another Lasix shot. He remained in the hospital for three days.

Two weeks later I returned to work. I had no choice. We needed the double insurance coverage. My insurance company covered what the primary insurance didn't. A babysitter came to the house during the day and did the best she could. Usually it took forty-five minutes to feed Westley two ounces of milk, and then he often threw it up. He just wanted to stay in his swing and suck his pacifier.

Meanwhile, Erik was proving to be an easy baby. He was friendly and invariably smiling. He was progressing and gaining weight. Westley, on the other hand, was distant and cranky. He still often cried when we held him. Even though he remained a slow feeder, I felt reassured that the gavage feedings at night helped him. But one evening, the nurse again had trouble inserting the feeding tube, and Westley went back to the hospital for the third time. His liver had become enlarged again, and he needed another Lasix shot.

I went straight from work to the hospital to visit him, and one of the doctors came down from the NICU to pay me a visit. He seemed upset—with me. He told me the hospital was doing the same things the nurses at our house were doing, and the problem was mine. He felt we needed family counseling. I knew the doctor was wrong, but I was too emotionally exhausted to argue, so I remained silent.

Westley came back home, and it remained pretty much the same story. He would do okay for a few days, then slide back downhill. He was rigid and did not want to be held.

A nurse came to the house one evening at eight o'clock and tried to insert the feeding tube. Again and again, Westley arched his back and screamed, and the nurse couldn't insert the tube. She called another nurse for assistance—who couldn't insert the tube, either. They called the supervising nurse, and she was unsuccessful as well. By 11:00 p.m., Westley had been screaming for three hours. My husband asked the nurses to stop trying and sent them home. I admitted him to the hospital for the fourth time.

The following day I left work early to visit Westley. I kept remembering what the doctor from the NICU had said to me. I was hurt and angry. By the time I arrived at the hospital, I was defensive. As I approached Westley's room, I heard him screaming. I walked in his room, and the nurse looked frantic. She could not insert the feeding tube. She looked up at me and asked, "How do you do it?" I told her the nurses coming to our house were having the same problem. She took a business card out of her pocket and handed it to me. "Call this nurse," she said. "She specializes in high-risk infant care. Her name is Junelle Pearson."

After Westley was released from the hospital, we hired Junelle to take over his care. Junelle could see that we were a family in crisis. She was a smart, warm, supportive person with a positive attitude. When Westley cried, she rocked him, holding him in a fetal position. He was rigid. Westley had been so premature, Junelle explained, that he "missed" being curled up in the womb, where developmental fine-tuning takes place. She also noticed that the previous nursing agency was using an adult-size gavage tube, which was trapping air in his stomach. That mistake explained his crankiness and why he fought so hard against the gavage tube. Fortunately, Junelle came with a supply of infant-size gavage tubes. The next morning Westley woke up smiling.

I had a good feeling about Junelle. She could feel when his liver was enlarged so we could take him to the pediatrician's office for a Lasix shot, which prevented him from being hospitalized again.

Every night Junelle held Westley in a fetal position, and she rocked him for several minutes as he cried. She bent his legs and arms to loosen him up. In about a week he was no longer sobbing when we held him, and shortly after that he was crying to be held. We could finally bond. It was hard enough dealing with his physical health, but I was equally concerned about his emotional development. At about eight months he began to emerge from his shell. Not only did he make great eye contact, but he also looked as if he were looking right into my soul. There was something deep about this baby.

Junelle often discussed early intervention with us. She said premature infants are at high risk for being delayed, and they need to be enrolled in infant/toddler programs to help them with their development. Because of my babies' low birth weights, their risk of becoming developmentally disabled, and Westley's hyaline membrane disease, they qualified for state funding from the Department of Developmental Services. Services are provided through state-operated developmental centers and contracts with nonprofit agencies called regional centers. A caseworker from the Westside Regional Center came to our house to evaluate the kids and suggested services that would benefit them.

Chris and I were excited by the boys' developmental improvements. Even though Erik was premature, he was crawling, sitting up, and walking by the time he turned one. When Westley's swing stopped rocking, his brother pushed the swing again. They had a special bond.

Westley continued to need an occasional Lasix shot for water retention, as well as his other diuretic medicines. Nonetheless, we were thrilled with the progress he had made. Not all was well, however. During an appointment at the pediatrician's office, the doctor noticed Westley's stiffness and told us he was at high risk for developing cerebral palsy. It was a prediction I could not accept. I automatically went into denial. (Luckily, his prediction turned out not to be true; two and a half years later, a pediatrician would rule out cerebral palsy.)

Junelle continued to work with Westley by helping him roll over and push himself up. She was relentless in talking to us about early intervention, even though many doctors adopt the "let's wait and see" philosophy because they don't want to alarm the parents unnecessarily. Yet the first three years of life can have the greatest impact on development. The brain is 90 percent developed by the time a child turns three.

Junelle was vindicated when the *Los Angeles Times* ran a front-page article titled "Early Help Cuts Premature Babies' Risks, Study Finds." The article reported that 250,000 babies are born underweight in the United States each year. Those children who received medical and family support as well as early education enjoyed significant increases in their developmental potential and quality of life. The nation-

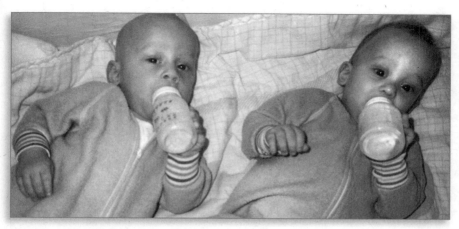

Westley and Erik at twelve months

wide study of 985 premature, low-birth-weight babies found that those who were enrolled in an early education program in the first three years of life scored up to thirteen points higher than others on IQ tests and were half as likely to develop behavioral problems.

As a new mother, I had no children to compare my children to—except each other. Erik and Westley had such different personalities. Erik was the party boy, always smiling, playful, and inquisitive. Westley was the serious one. He seemed to be the thinker—even though I frequently observed Westley banging his head against the back of his highchair while he ate his meals. They both talked in their own language that nobody could understand. I was told that twins often create a language of their own and that it was not unusual for preemies to have speech delays. I assumed the boys would catch up sooner rather than later.

Westley started to take his first steps at fourteen and a half months. He was clumsy and had a tendency to fall and bump into things. One day, while we were outside on the patio, he fell, smashed his forehead, and developed an egg-size bump. I cried harder than Westley. I kept ice on it as much as he would allow me to. Not long after that episode, he fell and received a bad cut above his eyelid. It needed seven stitches.

At Junelle's urging, I took him to UCLA to be evaluated by pediatrician Judy Howard. She observed Westley for several minutes, then turned to me and said, "What a fascinating child." She found him stubborn, controlling, and intelligent. It was her sense that he was quite bright, and because he'd been sick for so long, he developed head banging as a way to soothe himself. She did not observe any autistic-like features or mental retardation and recommended a preschool toddler program once he turned eighteen months old.

Dr. Howard also evaluated Erik and concluded that his physical and neurological exams were normal. His rate of development was average or above average

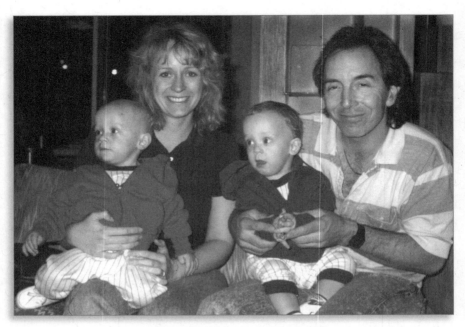

Deborah and Chris, with Westley (left) and Erik at eighteen months

for a toddler who'd been born preterm, though he had some fine-motor skill delays in how he used his hands to work with puzzles. Erik was easygoing and delightful, Dr. Howard said, and he would also benefit from a toddler preschool.

The boys continued to talk in their shared language. I occasionally discerned a recognizable word, such as "dog" or "ball." When Erik was eighteen months old, I heard him say, "Bye-bye, Dada" as my husband pulled out of the driveway. I was thrilled.

One day, the boys' aunt came by and gave them a puzzle, designated for ages three to five. I thanked her but explained the children wouldn't be able to put together a puzzle that advanced. Erik promptly dumped all the pieces out and completed it in seconds.

Erik was quite a climber, too, and it wasn't long before he was climbing out of his crib. I was concerned that his brother would try to copy him.

Westley was beginning to thrive, and it appeared that the medical crisis was over. It was time to say good-bye to Junelle. My husband and I were grateful to her, for she saved all of us from many potential catastrophes. One of the greatest gifts she gave was her belief in me. I was strong, she told me, and a good mother. It was challenging enough being a mother of twins. Having twins with special needs put motherhood on a completely different level. We needed all the help and encouragement we could get. Junelle was heaven sent. If not for her, my kids could have easily fallen through the cracks.

Addressing their needs had proven costly. Thankfully, we had insurance. In adding up all the medical bills for Westley in his first eighteen months of life, we arrived at a cost of about $450,000. That included the NICU, four hospitalizations, and in-home nursing. Erik's tab from the NICU was around $85,000.

The Terrible Twos Times Two

When the boys were twenty-seven months old, I stopped working and stayed at home to care for them. Westley was thriving, and double insurance was no longer a necessity. Even though their language was delayed, they certainly knew their numbers and letters, thanks to a heavy dosage of Sesame Street. Erik could identify numbers up to twenty-five.

Nap time was always a challenge. One afternoon, I put the boys down for a nap; about fifteen minutes later I heard laughter coming from their room. I opened the door and saw that Erik had taken off all his clothes. Westley was standing on his bookcase with his diaper off, pulling his shirt over his head, ready to fall and hit his head again. They had ripped all the pages out of their Little Golden Books. I was in for a double dosage of the terrible twos.

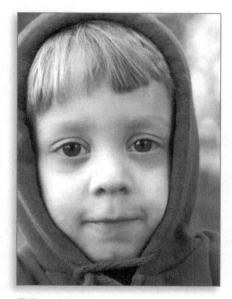

Erik at two years

Erik loved *National Geographic.* The living room floor was always covered with magazines. He pulled them out of the living room bookcase and opened them to the elephant pictures. Later, Erik developed a new fascination: dinosaurs. When he spoke, I couldn't understand him, but I knew he was talking about dinosaurs.

I took the boys to be evaluated at the Westside Regional Center. I knew they had language delays; however, I was surprised to learn that Westley's language skills were at a fourteen-and-a-half-month level. His social skills were at a twelve-and-a-half-month level. He was more than one year delayed. His fine motor, gross motor, and cognitive skills were eight months behind. Erik's language skills were at a fourteen-and-a-half-month level. His social skills were at a twenty-month level. His fine motor, gross motor, and cognitive skills were six months delayed.

At last I comprehended the importance of early intervention. Both boys began receiving weekly occupational therapy. They were also placed in an infant/toddler program for children at risk. It was a new program, and they were the first to be enrolled. They attended three days a week for three hours. When they began the program, they were not saying their own names. By the end of the first week, they were not only saying their own names but also each other's, though they continued to use their own private language.

The downside of the boys' being in the toddler program classroom was that they caught frequent infections. Erik had an ongoing ear infection, while Westley had frequent sinus and ear infections. Shortly after they turned two and a half they were on the antibiotic merry-go-round.

Infections aside, the boys made good progress in the toddler program, even though they continued to show global developmental delays. They were described as having difficulties in organization and behavior, particularly in distractibility and impulsivity, and poor registration and modulation of sensory input from their environment. They both had difficulties with oral motor control and fine motor skills.

I began hearing the professionals who worked with my children describe them with an unfamiliar diagnosis: pervasive developmental disorder. At the time I was clueless as to what it meant; I thought it was a professional term for being delayed. I later learned it was another term for autism. The boys' teacher eventually told me she thought they were both autistic when they began her program. Autistic or not, by the time the boys turned three, they were showing signs of attention deficit hyperactivity disorder (ADHD): distractibility, short attention span, and restlessness.

Preschool

Once the boys turned three, they no longer qualified for Regional Center state funding. It was time for the Los Angeles Unified School District to provide services for them. The Los Angeles Unified School District offered occupational therapy as well as an early education program.

The boys were enrolled in a special educational program with a small student population, one teacher, and an aide. The autistic label followed Erik because he was less interactive than his brother. He continued to speak in his own language and was withdrawn. He knew his numbers, letters, and colors; nevertheless, his vocabulary consisted of about twenty-five words. He continued to obsess about dinosaurs.

Westley also exhibited severe difficulties in receptive and expressive language. His words were unintelligible. I requested that the twins be placed in a classroom that was more language based. At three and a half years old, they were enrolled in an aphasia class. The class was small and taught by a speech therapist and an aide. The classroom consisted of children with significant language delays and high-functioning autism.

Erik's limited attention span and difficulty following directions continued to be a challenge, though he made progress in other areas. He played obsessively with dinosaurs, but he was beginning to make more eye contact with his teachers and his peers.

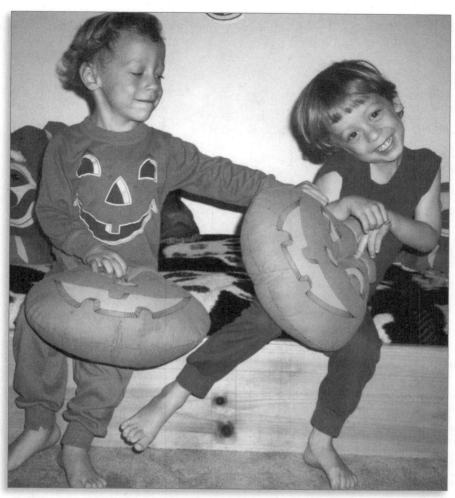

Westley and Erik at three years

Westley needed more help with his speech. He had low muscle tone, and his speaking was "slushy." While Erik had his dinosaurs, Westley showed unusual preoccupations with his shadow and looking at himself in the mirror. Both boys were described as spacing out at times and having difficulties staying on task. They continued to show poor muscle coordination and poor motor planning in activities. Fine motor skills remained elusive for both boys.

Because Erik was withdrawn and preoccupied with dinosaurs, we were advised to have him evaluated at the Regional Center for Autism when he turned four. Our case manager's instinct was that Erik probably didn't have autism, but it would be a good idea to have him evaluated to rule it out. While Westley was a

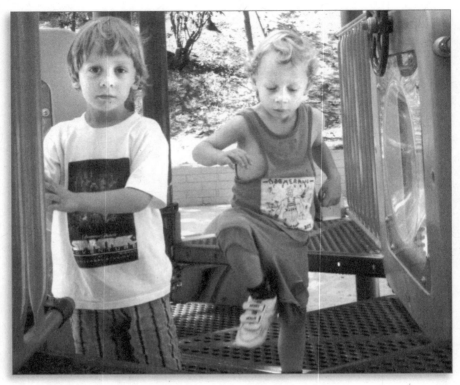

Erik and Westley at three years

bit on the eccentric side, no one felt that he was showing signs of autism, and he wasn't evaluated.

One month before Erik's fourth birthday, I took him to the Regional Center for his assessment. He lined up cars and dolls, a sign of autism. But he made eye contact with the examiner and used up to four words in a sentence. Her findings were that he was not autistic. She noted some distractibility and that he was immature for his age.

We had a pony birthday party for the boys to celebrate their fourth birthday. Usually the boys were friendly and active when we had friends over. This time Erik was unusually withdrawn; he went to a corner to play by himself. I was beginning to wonder whether this was the autistic behavior that his teachers were referring to. As it turned out he had an ear infection brewing and did not feel well. He became more social after being on antibiotics for a few days.

The boys were evaluated by their occupational therapist, who concluded that their occupational therapy should be increased to two times a week. They were given the Peabody Development Test, which evaluated their fine motor skills. Westley was more than two years delayed.

When Westley was retested at four and a half years old, it was discovered that his motor skills were at a twenty-five-month level. He had insufficient strength to put interlocking blocks together. He was unable to write his first name and was always the last one to complete a task. He was described as sometimes being in a "dreamlike state."

Erik's fine motor skills were at a thirty-one-month level. He could not cut with scissors. A few isolated skills were tested at a forty-eight-month level. Erik knew numbers up to fifty. Meanwhile, he continued to talk nonstop about dinosaurs.

I dreaded taking the boys to the market with me. They fought over who would sit in the cart seat. It was too intense to take them out. Westley liked to go to the cereal aisle, and Erik searched for dinosaur toys. Wherever we went, we were noticed because of the boys' high energy level. Usually people would be more accepting of them once they realized they were twins.

The boys and I had repeated respiratory infections. Erik and Westley visited the pediatrician at least once a month. We were all developing allergies to some of the antibiotics. I had a permanent ear or respiratory infection. My energy was low. I used to attend an aerobics class, but now I could barely complete four minutes on a stationary bicycle.

At about this time, Chris and I decided to move to a new house, right behind a good elementary school. While we were packing up the house, we moved our bed away from the wall and discovered black mold growing everywhere. I wondered whether it had been behind our chronic infections. I was glad we were moving.

The boys were excited about the new house. Chris and I were, too; it was our hope that Erik and Westley would be able to attend a regular classroom at the neighborhood school by first grade. They were still more than a year away from starting kindergarten.

In the new house I tried to keep the boys busy while I unpacked. I brought their little table and chairs into my room and told Erik to draw some pictures. A few minutes later I suggested that he write the alphabet. He replied, "I just did." I was surprised that I could read every letter. Erik's fine motor skills were catching up.

The boys went outside to play on the back porch. I heard them talking through the wall. "Hey, Westley!" Erik said. "Don't tell Mom, but look at what I'm doing." I stopped unpacking and went to see what Erik did not want me to see. He had dumped dirt and small rocks into his play workbench sink. It was a mess. I asked him not to bring dirt and rocks up to the porch. He replied in a matter-of-fact voice, "Those are dinosaur fossils, Mom." At moments like these, Erik reminded me of Dennis the Menace.

Before he got out of bed in the morning, we could hear him loudly lecturing, "The triceratops lived 100 million years ago." I found it interesting to observe a boy who, despite a significant expressive language delay, became so articulate when identifying all the dinosaurs and the facts relevant to them.

Although they could both be charming children, they were also at times difficult. Westley was throwing tantrums, and they were both rebellious. At four and a half, they appeared stuck in the terrible twos. It was time for me to find professional help for them.

I found a psychologist who worked with children with behavioral problems. I told her that I thought both boys exhibited ADHD symptoms and that some professionals had found evidence of high-functioning autism, particularly in Erik's case. He was still obsessed with dinosaurs and often acted as though he was not hearing what people said to him. But I made it quite clear that I did not believe that my kids were autistic.

In evaluating Erik, the psychologist found him to be delayed overall by six months. His strengths: working with blocks, drawing, recognizing colors, using and understanding numbers, accepting his body image, and matching. His weaknesses: fine and gross motor skills, auditory memory, expressive and receptive language, play, and social skills. His spontaneous language often consisted of engaging the examiner in, not surprisingly, a conversation about dinosaurs. He also sometimes acted as though he did not hear the examiner's requests; he isolated himself from her and continued to play with his dinosaurs. When she examined the boys playing together with their toys, Erik did not interact with his brother.

In evaluating Westley, the psychologist determined he was overall a year delayed. Color labeling, number concepts, and matching were among his strengths; his weaknesses were in the areas of drawing, body image, visual memory, expressive language, play, social development, and gross motor skills. He also exhibited difficulty paying attention and poor impulse control. Westley became frustrated when he could not do simple tasks; he would then throw tantrums. His behavior was becoming aggressive, and he had quite a temper. He flung his toys and hit his brother—yet when he wanted to, Westley could be a charming child.

The psychologist was helpful in her suggestions about disciplining them. We began to create "reward charts" at the end of the day. When the boys earned enough stickers they would receive a small toy. I also began implementing timeouts, which proved more effective with Westley than Erik. Erik could be very belligerent. Every time I took the boys out, Erik would demand that I buy him a toy. When I refused, he would throw a tantrum. Westley, on the other hand, rarely asked me to buy him anything.

The boys continued in their aphasia class and were making good progress; however, we were still coming down with frequent respiratory infections and taking antibiotics.

We lived across the street from a small park with playground equipment for young children. The park provided a great opportunity for the boys, now five years old, to work on their gross motor skills. But Westley became frustrated with his lack of coordination. He tended to be accident prone. He watched children much younger than himself climb the circle bars, while he could barely climb them at all.

Meanwhile, Erik was becoming more social. He would seek out new playmates every time we went to the park and was becoming a real boy's boy. Erik had a strong curiosity and enjoyed exploring. He was beginning to speak more

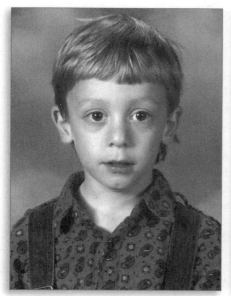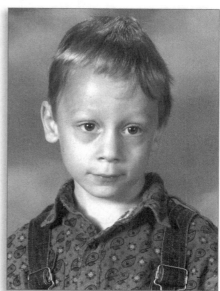

Erik and Westley in preschool

appropriately for his age. He continued to obsess on dinosaurs—and developed a new preoccupation: Legos.

Westley was very serious and would usually like to be in the backyard. He played mostly with his stuffed animals and toy telephones, and would often have conversations with an imaginary friend.

The one thing I knew for sure was that I did not have run-of-the-mill kids.

When they turned five and a half, I had the boys reevaluated by the psychologist. She reported that Erik continued to use his own language to initiate interactions with others. He made repeated statements, and she said his voice was unusual, distinguished by a mildly hollow tone. But he was making progress and was only seven months delayed overall. She did not come out and say that Erik was autistic; however, she hinted at it. Almost all the professionals who worked with him reported some autistic symptoms. I thought that if he were autistic he would always show the symptoms. The only time I would observe autistic behaviors—such as being withdrawn and aloof—was when he was coming down with an infection. I suspected that many of the professionals thought I was in denial, that I would not be able to face the truth—that both of my sons were autistic.

In evaluating Westley, the psychologist found him to be very charming and engaging. He had made great progress in some areas, such as auditory memory. Like Erik, he used his own language to initiate conversations. His language was both delayed and idiosyncratic. He also had a lateral lisp. The psychologist suggested that Ritalin could help Westley focus on tasks and materials, sustain both visual and auditory attention, and screen out exogenous stimuli.

When I told Chris that the psychologist had recommended medication for Westley, he became upset. "No way is he going to be taking Ritalin," Chris declared. I told Chris that I would have Westley examined by a psychiatrist. "Go ahead," he replied, "but my answer will remain the same."

I took Westley to the psychiatrist. He gave me the Conners Teacher Questionnaire, enumerating the different symptoms of ADHD as a checklist to be filled out by his teacher. She checked off a slew of symptoms. Westley was restless in a "squirmy" sense, had a short attention span, and was excitable and impulsive much of the time. The teacher hoped he would go on Ritalin. So did the psychiatrist. At this point, a psychologist, a psychiatrist, and a teacher had concluded that Westley should be medicated—but my husband was resolute. "Perhaps some children do need it," he said, "but it would not help Westley."

At the Individualized Education Program meeting, the teachers recommended that Westley remain in the aphasia class. Due to the boys' gross motor skill delays, they were enrolled in an adaptive physical education course, geared toward children whose gross motor skills were behind and for those with disabilities. The boys continued to receive occupational therapy in school and once a week in the clinic.

Erik's gross motor skills remained about one year behind. He was making very good progress in other areas. By the time he was five and a half his fine motor skills were at his age level. He continued to fixate on dinosaurs, in addition to a new interest—the color red. He was described as having a good self-image and was making progress in his social skills. The major concern was that he liked to tease other children and test the limits of the classroom rules. At the Individualized Education Program meeting, the teachers recommended for the next year that Erik be mainstreamed into a regular kindergarten class for two and a half hours and then return to the aphasia class for speech therapy.

Kindergarten

I was a little nervous and excited about Erik being mainstreamed into kindergarten. He was going from a small class to an overcrowded one. His attention disorder presented a challenge for the teacher, and his disruptive behavior persisted.

One day, Erik came home from school with a distressing note from his teacher. The kindergarten class had worked hard in recycling cans and paper, earning enough money to buy good scissors for the classroom. Erik destroyed the scissors by covering them with glue. The teacher was unable to remove the glue and sent us the scissors in a bag, so we could see them.

I decided I should go and observe Erik in school so I could see what was going on firsthand. I arrived at his class while the children were at recess. When they returned, Erik walked right past me—he didn't notice I was in the classroom. All the children sat down, and Erik was in the back. While the teacher was talking, Erik flipped through big pictures hanging on the easel. The teacher twice asked him to stop.

I knew Erik was a handful for his teacher. I could see the stress on her face in dealing with him. He always required adult supervision to get back on task. I felt guilty and frustrated about the situation. And I really felt bad for the teacher.

Meanwhile, Westley was making good academic progress. His reading, math, and spelling skills were at his age level. He was described as being friendly, and he got along well with his peers. His two favorite things to do during free time at school were to play house in the little house in the schoolyard and dress up in costumes. Unfortunately, his fine and gross motor skills remained delayed, and his attention disorder was an ongoing issue. He frequently looked in the mirror at his reflection or watched his shadow.

When the boys turned six, I had them reevaluated by the psychologist. Erik was given the Peabody Individual Achievement Test, which indicated that he'd made great progress in many areas and was demonstrating capabilities at an early-to mid-kindergarten level. His most significant areas of weakness continued to be in behavior, language, and gross motor skills. The psychologist noted that he was wiggly and fidgety and, at times, would not remain seated. She said he had symptoms of ADHD. The psychologist recommended that Erik be mainstreamed into a regular first grade class in the coming year, with speech and language therapy and adaptive physical education to help him improve his gross motor skills. Finally, she used the M word; she suggested medicine to target his distractibility and hyperactive behaviors.

Westley's evaluation was much more alarming. He had made little progress since the last test. His greatest strengths were in body image, auditory memory, and number skills. His areas of weaknesses included fine motor, gross motor, and puzzle skills, as well as sustained attention to tasks, strategy development, and frustration tolerance. Overall, Westley was delayed by eighteen months.

The psychologist went on to say that Westley exhibited a complex fantasy life. He had brought a stuffed animal with him, which he put down for a nap during the session. After the testing, he related to the psychologist a dream that he said the stuffed animal had while they were working. The dream involved his family members and the circus. She found this behavior to be odd. He repeatedly asked her where Erik and I went during the testing, even though he knew the answer. She recommended that Westley continue in the aphasia class for the following year, with occupational therapy and adaptive physical education—and that, like Erik, he should be considered for a medicine trial.

I knew it was going to be futile to discuss the medication issue with Chris. He strongly opposed Ritalin. I had mixed feelings about it. In doing research, I discovered that Ritalin (generically known as methylphenidate) suppressed appetite and growth—and my kids were already only between the tenth and twenty-fifth percentile for their height and weight. I also learned that some of the side effects of Ritalin were motor tics and a set of behaviors comparable to Tourette's syndrome. Westley already had recurring facial tics, and I worried that Ritalin may possibly exacerbate his Tourette's-like behaviors. And I was confused why doctors were recommending Ritalin when they knew that Westley had facial tics.

The kids had been through enough because of their premature birth. They were both bright, and it was my husband's gut feeling that they would both be okay without taking drugs. On the other hand, I was the one who was with them most of the time. Raising twins with an attention disorder was stressful to the point that it had an impact on my health. I was always sick with ear infections, bronchitis, headaches, and chronic fatigue. I felt pressure from teachers always complaining about my kids' hyperactivity.

The psychologist could not understand Chris's aversion to Ritalin; it had been around forever, and millions of children were taking it. "Just try it for a few weeks and see if you see an improvement," she said. Chris told me to get a second opinion.

I took them to another psychiatrist. It had been raining hard that day, and the boys were more hyper than usual. We were on the second floor, on our way to the doctor's office, when Erik disappeared. All of a sudden I heard screaming and crying echoing throughout the courtyard. He was lying on the ground outside. I thought he had fallen from the second floor. He had actually walked down the stairs and slipped. He was fine. I was not. I was ready to put them on Ritalin.

The psychiatrist strongly suggested that Erik needed medication. In observing Westley, she saw some hints of Tourette's as well as an attention deficit.

Because I knew Chris would still object to medication, I insisted that he have a private session with the psychiatrist to discuss it. I was hoping she would be able to get through to him.

When Chris came home that night, the first words out of his mouth were, "They are not going to take Ritalin. And if you put them on it, I will divorce you."

"What do you suggest we do?" I asked.

"You have been looking into alternative medicine," he answered. "Try to treat it naturally."

My mother had been visiting us, and she told me about a book called *Is This Your Child?* by Doris Rapp, MD (Harper Paperbacks, 1991). The book linked allergies to hyperactivity, behavior issues, and learning disabilities. My mother told me that my kids looked allergic. She mentioned that they both had dark circles under their eyes. Certainly, something was wrong; it didn't make sense that the boys and I were fighting one infection after another or that we were on antibiotics more often than not. I decided to take them to an allergist.

The allergist noted that both boys appeared allergic. She observed water in Erik's ears. He had frequent ear infections, nasal congestion, and bronchitis. As it turned out, Erik had a severe dust-mite allergy. He also was allergic to mold, cats, several weeds, trees, and grasses.

Westley's examination was more alarming. The allergist detected a wheeze and diagnosed him as asthmatic. He also suffered from frequent sinusitis, ear infections, and headaches. At different times of the year, he would blink his eyes and clear his throat frequently. The allergist ordered a scratch prick test. Westley tested positive for allergies to cats and mold.

We bought a HEPA filter for the boys' bedroom to control dust and mold, and then put dust covers over their mattresses. They had allergy injections two times a week. It was no picnic taking them for their shots. They would rebel by misbehaving. Erik would frequently leave the waiting room and wander around the hallway, while Westley would switch the light on and off in the waiting room. I found myself constantly apologizing for their behavior. The more patients in the waiting room, the more obnoxious they would be; the boys always loved an audience. After an allergy shot they were supposed to wait twenty to thirty minutes before we left, to make sure they had no reaction to the injection. I always found myself cutting out a few minutes early because of their behavior. I bribed them in the hopes they'd behave—I took them for fast food or bought them a toy. I did just about everything, except put them on Ritalin.

The allergist checked the boys frequently to observe how the allergy injections and other measures were working. Erik still had fluid in his ears. The lack of response frustrated all of us. It seemed as if Erik had a permanent ear infection.

I inquired about alternative medicine. The doctors I had been using were wary of alternative approaches and cautioned me to be very careful.

My first step on the alternative path led me to a chiropractor. In researching alternative medicine, I had learned that an aligned spine allows the nervous system to work optimally and can help the immune system function at a higher level, thereby keeping the body healthy. Neal Snyder understood and sympathized with my kids' situation. He found several misalignments in their spines, and the boys began receiving regular chiropractic treatments.

Meanwhile, my energy level was totally depleted. I was a full-time, stay-at-home mother, and I was too exhausted to volunteer at my kids' school. As soon as they left for school, I would go right back to bed and nurse an ear infection, bronchitis, or a headache. I was also experiencing vertigo.

The boys continued to be out of control when I took them for their allergy shots. After six months of chasing them around the doctor's office and always trying to explain why my kids acted the way they did, I gave up. I had no more energy. I did not care what people thought anymore. I was sure it was obvious that my children had special needs; so be it.

We also had many wonderful moments with our kids. When I took the boys to the park one day, a mother came up to me—to praise Erik. Erik had noticed her daughter crying; he then sat down next to the little girl, put his arm around her, and told her it was okay and that he would share his toys with her. I wish all the professionals who thought he was autistic could have witnessed that moment.

The boys were very affectionate and often played well together. Westley loved dressing up in his old Halloween costumes and playing make-believe. One day he would be Peter Pan and the next, a Power Ranger. He loved Michael Jackson's music and wanted to dance like him. It was a great challenge, thanks to his poor gross motor skills. He would become especially frustrated while attempting the moonwalk. No matter how many times he tried to get the movements down, he couldn't do it.

First Grade

The school bus picked up Westley every day to take him to his new school. A speech pathologist and an assistant taught his aphasia class. His teacher was quite an inspiration to Westley. When he came home from school, he would drag a small table from the living room into his bedroom and pretend to be a teacher. He wrote down all his imaginary pupils' names and put grades on their papers. In the course of his playing he managed to complete his homework. In no time he was performing academically at his age level or above, though his gross and fine motor skills remained delayed.

Erik attended the elementary school behind our house. He was mainstreamed into a regular first grade with twenty-nine students. Two-thirds of the students were boys. Academically he was performing from average to above for his age. Erik made friends easily and became popular with the boys' clique. Unfortunately, his teacher found his nonstop talking to be a problem. He lacked verbal self-control and often jumped out of his seat.

His obsession with dinosaurs persisted—he often played with the variety of Transformer toys that metamorphosed into dinosaurs. His interest would make

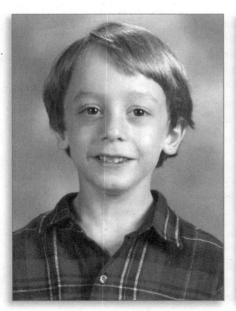
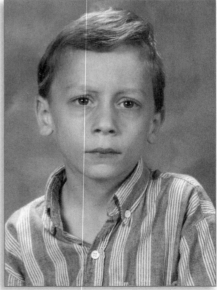

Erik and Westley in first grade

its way into his schoolwork. When the teacher wrote a phrase about Franklin and Eleanor Roosevelt on the chalkboard and asked students to respond with an appropriate drawing, Erik drew a stegosaurus with an American flag covering half of its body. The drawing showed natural talent and imagination.

Westley's therapist went to observe him at school. She said he was standing in line with the other children when he suddenly started to twitch and jerk his head around, watching his shadow. I laughed; I knew he was doing his impression of Michael Jackson. Unfortunately, he was calling negative attention to himself. The other children would make fun of him, and he would become upset. Westley was a worrier, but he was also very sensitive and caring. The adults really liked him because he was different and an interesting child to watch. He was often described as walking to the beat of his own drum. Whenever we went into a store, he would find a mirror to look at his reflection. This had been going on since he was a toddler.

Erik had good and bad days at school. He needed a lot of help staying on task. When he became too much to handle, the teacher would send him to the other first grade class until he could contain himself. His teacher said that, at one point, he was crawling on the floor, imitating a lizard.

After hearing about this, the psychologist couldn't understand why we wouldn't put Erik on Ritalin. I knew I had to do something. I was burned out going to doctors all the time. Chris was working twelve hours a day, often six days a week. On his one day off, he would be an enormous help; however, it was never enough.

Exhausted, I went to the doctor. I was diagnosed with Hashimoto's thyroiditis, an autoimmune disease causing an underactive thyroid. The diagnosis explained why I was chronically tired. The thyroid medicine helped take the edge off, but I was still tired and had frequent headaches and infections.

We had good insurance coverage; nevertheless, the deductibles, along with all of our other medical needs, were taking their toll on our finances. Chris believed that we were spending too much money on doctors and allergy medicines, with little progress. At this point, I decided to look into alternative medicine beyond chiropractic. If my husband wouldn't allow the kids to go on Ritalin, then I would try the alternative path, even though our insurance would not cover most of it.

My chiropractor suggested that I take my kids to see a doctor who specializes in traditional Chinese medicine (TCM). I visited him first to check him out and see if he could really help us. He took me off all dairy products and sugar and gave me awful-tasting Chinese herbs to take every day. I knew my boys would not put up with the herbs and would resist the dietary restrictions. They loved dairy products, and Erik was addicted to milk.

Regardless, after one month I began to feel better and the ear infections and vertigo vanished—and I decided it might be worthwhile to take the kids to see him. He examined both of them and requested we remove dairy and sugar from their diets. He allowed them one serving of fruit a day. I managed, by some miracle, to get them off dairy, and I reduced their sugar intake as well. I began buying soymilk, though they didn't care for it.

Through this doctor I learned that cow's milk and other dairy products are toxic to humans—cow's milk is designed for calves, not people. More than thirty years of research shows that cow's milk is connected to colic; ear infections; allergies; asthma; chronic sinusitis; menstrual problems; lung, breast, ovarian, and uterine cancer; heart disease; and diabetes in children. Dairy products have antibiotic and pesticide residues, which also damage the immune system. I didn't want to expose my family to any more pesticides, so I began to buy organic produce at the farmer's market.

When Erik's allergist examined him a month later, she noticed that the fluid in his ears had vanished. He was no longer getting ear infections. It appeared that a dairy allergy had been the problem. His teacher and I could see a difference. He still talked too much but was beginning to make a real effort to improve his behavior. Convinced that dairy should be permanently removed from my children's diets, I began to purchase calcium-fortified juices and calcium supplements.

Dairy allergies cost my family countless infections and visits to the doctor's office. Not one of our doctors ever suspected that dairy products were the cause of Erik's or my persistent ear infections. They'd just continued to prescribe antibiotics.

We did not continue to see the TCM doctor because his office was too far away. He'd gotten us on the right path though, and I was grateful for that. I had many revelations about Erik's autistic symptoms and strongly believed that the chronic fluid in his ears had contributed to his autistic-like behavior.

Erik began to complain profusely about being pulled out of class for adaptive physical education. He wanted to be in regular P.E. with all his buddies. The adaptive P.E. teacher tested Erik and found his gross motor skills were at his proper age level, and he was placed in regular physical education classes. His speech had also improved, and he was becoming quite articulate.

Chris insisted that it was time for Westley to be mainstreamed into second grade. Academically he was flying. He was a natural speller and received 100 percent on all of his spelling tests. His expressive language had improved, although his speech remained slushy, due to low muscle tone. His vocabulary and reading skills were above the levels expected for his age, and his tics were diminishing.

He remained somewhat eccentric, and we hoped that being with mainstream children would help him catch up socially. He would need to continue in adaptive P.E., speech therapy, and occupational therapy to address his fine motor skills. Considering everything he had been through, we were very pleased with his progress.

Second Grade

My husband's hunches were correct. Westley made a smooth transition to full inclusion into second grade. He went from a class of eight students to twenty-nine students with one teacher. His academic skills were above average. His handwriting remained very poor. His obsession with Michael Jackson was beginning to fade. Star Wars was his new thing—he wanted to be Luke Skywalker.

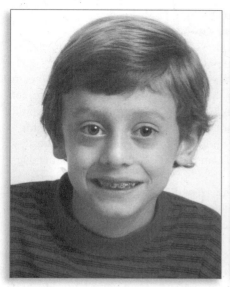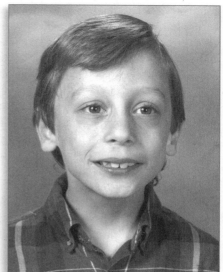

Erik and Westley in second grade

Erik made good academic progress and remained popular among his peers. The biggest obstacle was his motor mouth. The teacher would leave messages on the answering machine saying that Erik's talking had advanced to a new level. He still had poor impulse control. The only service he was receiving at that time was a full-inclusion teacher. She would visit the classroom once a week to check on his progress and offer suggestions to the teacher.

The school principal said that my boys were the perfect students for full inclusion. They were overly qualified for special education, however, and still had to be monitored to make sure they were making progress. We were fortunate to be receiving so many services.

One day, Westley got into trouble in the schoolyard at lunchtime. He was climbing up on the table with the other boys when a mother who had volunteered for yard duty asked them to get off the table. The boys called her names, and Westley told her she stank. They were taken to the principal's office. The kids stayed after school to write an apology. The teacher said that Westley was truly remorseful and quite shaken by what he had done. He was having a hard time making friends and would hang around the kids who tended to get into mischief. They were the only ones who would accept him.

I continued to have second thoughts about Ritalin. I kept in touch with the psychiatrist who had originally diagnosed Westley with ADHD. He said as long as he was making academic progress, he would be okay not taking Ritalin.

Adults enjoyed Westley because he was unique, unusually sensitive, and insightful. I was amazed at the questions he would ask me, such as whether the universe could move. I was clueless as to how to answer him. I only knew that I wasn't asking those kinds of questions when I was in second grade!

The boys still received allergy shots once a week. Erik was beginning to mature and didn't give me such a hard time. Westley was another story. He was very defiant and would not go to the nurse when it was his turn for a shot. He would scream when he received his injection. Back in the waiting room, he continued to act out. Once we got home and he had calmed down, I would ask him why he would act this way every time he received a shot. His reply would be that he couldn't help it and that he didn't want to go anymore. At times it seemed that Westley really didn't care what people thought of him. Usually he was sweet and engaging, but he was also unpredictable.

When Westley reached the end of the second grade, everyone was pleased with his academic progress, though his teacher said that he remained socially awkward. It was difficult for children and adults to understand him. He was still uncoordinated and would have to remain in adaptive physical education. He continued to have sinus infections but not as frequently as before.

The boys played well together most of the time, except Westley would scratch, bite, kick, or hit his brother when he became angry. They were both into Star Wars and loved action figures. Westley loved his toys too much—he would chew on them. Concerned about possible lead exposure, I called the toy companies, who assured me that their products were lead free. Nonetheless, I was constantly asking Westley to get toys out of his mouth.

He also resisted using his utensils at mealtime. I often wondered whether his low muscle tone was preventing him from using a fork or knife. He would finger feed himself all his peas, rice, cereal, meat, and pasta. The only time he would use a spoon was when he was eating yogurt. All his books would be smeared with barbeque sauce or whatever he had just eaten.

I was tired of nagging my kids or telling them what they were doing wrong, and I probably let too many things slide with regard to their poor daily habits. I was told to choose my battles wisely. When they did something right, I went overboard praising them. I didn't want them to suffer poor self-esteem.

When the boys were in second grade, the state of California started to use the Stanford 9 Achievement Test for evaluating students' academic skills, identifying where they stood compared to other children their age across the country. The boys' test results were weak in some areas, but overall, they were in the ballpark for the average child. Westley excelled in spelling, where his scores ranked in the eighty-second percentile. Erik was making good progress, with age-appropriate scores in all areas.

Third Grade

The full-inclusion teacher would visit the boys' classrooms once a week to monitor their progress. Westley continued with a full range of services to meet his needs. An occupational therapist worked with him at school to address his poor handwriting skills, and he continued with speech therapy and adaptive physical education.

Even though Westley was making good academic progress, I saw a regression in his handwriting. It was getting much worse. He was also becoming more aggressive toward Erik. He often scratched, hit, kicked, or bit him.

Erik still had some behavioral issues of his own, including poor impulse control. But he was always happy and appeared to have high self-esteem. He had many friends in and out of school and was quite social. Westley, on the other hand, was having a challenging time with other children. He frequently ate lunch alone. Erik told me that he would see his brother walking around in circles and talking to himself. Sometimes it would appear that he was talking to a tree. Kids were beginning to make fun of him. Erik would sometimes ask his brother to join him for lunch, but Westley would decline. He wanted to make his own friends.

Every week we took the boys out to dinner at a restaurant—where Westley generally went out of his way to embarrass us. He would yell or kick his chair. The yelling and poor attitude would begin on the way to the restaurant. Once dinner came, we would all manage to calm down and enjoy our meal. His father would ask him, "Whatever happened to the old Westley?"

I usually refused to be drawn into Westley's dramatic scenes; I felt that by giving him too much attention I would add more fuel to the fire. Instead, we would take privileges away and give him timeouts. It would work for a day or two, but he continued to suffer from a lack of impulse control and often seemed agitated.

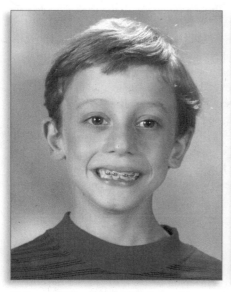 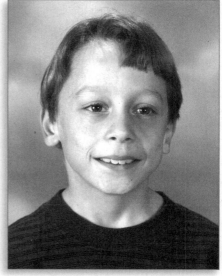

Erik and Westley in third grade

School was closed the day before Thanksgiving, and I had to take the boys on some errands. First, we went to the market to pick up the turkey. We were standing at the deli counter when Westley suddenly went ballistic on Erik. He started to strangle him and knocked him to the ground. You could see red fingerprints on Erik's neck. A woman standing at the deli counter witnessed the whole episode and appeared horrified. I got the boys out of the market as quickly as possible. On the way home I gave Westley a major tongue-lashing. I told him that when he got home he would spend the rest of the day cleaning his room, and that he did. He found long-lost toys, cleaned out his entire closet, and did an incredible job. Then he wrote his brother an apology.

As the school year progressed, Erik decided that he didn't want to do his homework anymore. He was constantly sneaking away from the table, and I would have to bring him back to task. Westley would rush through his homework, and it was impossible to read his handwriting.

It was an emotionally draining time. We had stopped seeing the psychologist—I was tired of being told to put my kids on Ritalin. And in addition to the challenge the boys presented on a daily basis, both of my husband's parents had passed away within nine months of each other.

When the boys were at the end of third grade, we had their Individualized Education Program meeting. Although it was recommended that Westley continue to receive all the supporting services already in place, the teacher reported he was showing substantial improvements, academically and socially. He was reading at his age level, with the more advanced group. He had established some friendships and shown growth in the classroom activities. Everyone felt that Westley had made progress—everyone except for me. I was seeing a decline, not only in his schoolwork but also his social skills. We received the results for the Stanford 9 Achievement Test series. He had made great progress in his reading skills, but he had dropped significantly in math and language. The most alarming result was his spelling score, which had dropped from the eighty-second percentile the year before to the twentieth percentile. I believed that he mistakenly checked off the wrong answers—his attention disorder was probably to blame.

Erik's teacher reported that he was at the appropriate grade level or slightly above. He was having a challenging time with his organization skills and didn't take his studies seriously. His behavior was somewhat immature and could be triggered by the poor behavior of others. But overall, the teacher was happy with Erik's progress and recommended that the full-inclusion teacher continue to monitor him in the fourth grade.

Fourth Grade

In the fourth grade, Erik got one of the most popular teachers—who gave relatively little homework. I was pleased, as I also needed a break. I could use a year off from constantly nagging Erik to do his homework. All that was required

THE MAIL ORDER CATALOG
PO Box 180
Summertown, TN 38483

The Mail Order Catalog carries the full line of books published by Book Publishing Company, plus many other alternative presses.

If you are interested in other fine books on vegetarian cooking, alternative health, or Native Americans, please mark your area of interest below and send for our catalog, or call 1-800-695-2241.

I would like to receive your book catalog on:

☐ Vegetarian cooking and nutrition
☐ Alternative health
☐ Native Americans

Name

Street or P.O. Box

City   **State**   **Zip**

Email address

www.healthy-eating.com • www.nativevoices.com

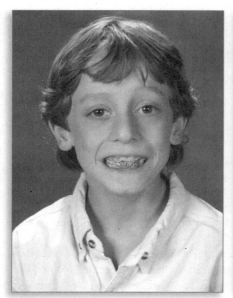 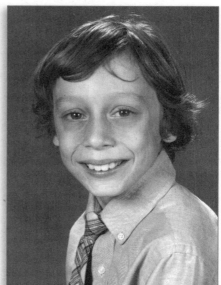

Erik and Westley in fourth grade

was one national current-event report each week. His teacher subscribed to a philosophy of teaching kids *how* to think instead of *what* to think. Erik continued to face the challenges of staying on task and using self-control. But he was becoming a real history buff and was making new friends.

Westley's fourth-grade teacher was perfect for him; her approach was both structured and creative. She was concerned for Westley socially. He had only one friend, and there was an excessive dependency on the friendship that led to many disappointments for him.

Academically, Westley's handwriting continued to be his biggest challenge. Nobody, including Westley, could read it. The occupational therapist would work with him by using a special pencil grip, but it didn't help much. He would rush through his assignments and sneak his work up to the teacher's desk when she was too busy to check it before accepting it. His poor handwriting hurt his math performance. He would not line up his numbers properly and, as a result, could not calculate the correct answer. Yet he was capable of understanding math concepts and had all the multiplication tables memorized.

Westley was also finding an outlet for his imagination and storytelling skills. He loved the creative-writing process, and his teacher saw some true natural talent.

Meanwhile, my health was beginning to improve. I used to go straight back to bed when my kids left for school. Now I was walking three miles every day and loving it. I had enough energy to volunteer at school and teach art history in both of my kids' classes.

Westley, on the other hand, was still experiencing sinus infections and often complained of headaches. He was receiving allergy injections every three weeks. He took a prescription allergy medicine, and used a nasal spray and an inhaler for his asthma every night before bed. His teacher felt he was having difficulty focusing much of the time. She suspected that he needed to be medicated for an attention disorder.

Oh, here we go again, I thought. I agreed there was a problem, but Ritalin was not the solution. I explained to her our concerns about Ritalin and added that her suggestion was nothing I hadn't heard many times before. Nothing else was said for a while. Even so, I was again having second thoughts about putting him on a trial run of Ritalin. I was very concerned for Westley—socially, as well as academically. I felt maybe the benefits would outweigh the liabilities of being medicated. I didn't want him to go through life as a failure with low self-esteem. I felt stuck between a rock and a hard place. I dealt with it by not dealing with it. I was burned out and needed a break from constant worry.

But it was hard not to worry about Westley. His teacher told me how the class would play a game to help the students memorize their science facts. When the students couldn't answer the question, she would say, "I am going to give the answer now." Westley would then yell, "Nooooo!" He received As on some tests and Ds on others. If his grade was low, he would become upset and walk around the classroom announcing his grade, saying, "I can't believe I got a D." He would try to calm himself down by telling the students that he was going to be okay. Yet I had never pressured my children to get As; knowing their challenges, I just wanted them to try their best.

One week, Westley had a sinus infection, which made it difficult for him to focus. His teacher was concerned, especially after she watched Westley while he thought he was sharpening his pencil in the pencil sharpener—he had neglected to put the pencil in it. His teacher said that he had been totally "spaced out." I felt pretty foolish myself and had no excuse for him. That night I told my husband about the incident. "No Ritalin," he insisted. I had recently read research about Ritalin causing cancer in laboratory animals and told Westley's teacher about the article. Her reply was, "Everything causes cancer."

Some people suggested biofeedback. Unfortunately, it was too expensive, and our insurance didn't cover it. I focused on doing what I could afford, especially when it came to what Westley and Erik ate. I visited the Santa Monica Farmer's Market every week to purchase organic fruit and vegetables, and the boys consumed no dairy and very little sugar. I decided to take wheat out of Westley's diet to see if there would be an improvement. He was such a trooper about giving up wheat, but we saw no difference after six weeks.

Meanwhile, Erik was flying academically. His only downfall was physical education; he was too busy socializing to follow the rules or participate enough. But he received mostly As and loved school, especially his history class. I enjoyed having him tell me about the history I could remember firsthand. He was learning about Vietnam, and I told him how my friends had driven from New Jersey to Washington, D.C., to protest against the war in the early 1970s. He asked if I had been a hippie, and I had a good laugh.

The full-inclusion teacher continued to visit both of the boys' classrooms once a week. She was impressed with Westley's sensitivity toward others and his brother. She didn't know how much he attacked Erik at home. Erik would tease him, and Westley would react by biting, hitting, kicking, or scratching him. Two hours later they would be playing with each other like nothing had happened. I knew most siblings behave in the same manner to varying degrees and assumed this behavior was more common with twins.

At the end of the year, we had their Individualized Education Program meeting to discuss the boys' progress. Erik's teacher reported that he had excelled academically in every subject and would receive straight As, though he was still talking too much in the classroom. "Never once did I yell, 'Shut up' to any of the students, until Erik," his teacher sighed. Erik had no other behavior problems, though, and did well socially. It was the consensus of the Individualized Education Program team that all special educational services be discontinued for him.

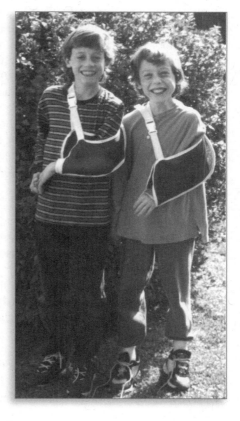

At Westley's Individualized Education Program meeting, the teacher said he had made progress in reading and creative writing. His teacher said that he "gives great details and is able to focus for longer periods of time." His math had improved as well. Science and social studies remained a challenge for him. Socially, he had a problem with interrupting other students. He would continue speech therapy, adaptive physical education, and occupational therapy. Overall he had a C-plus average.

We received the results of the Stanford 9 test over the summer. Erik performed well, except in spelling, where he had only scored in the thirty-second percentile. Erik was never a great speller.

Westley's Stanford 9 results were more upsetting—they had dropped substantially from the previous year. His total reading score was in the fifteenth percentile. His math results had dropped by ten percentile points, and his language score was only in the eighth percentile. The only area he excelled in was spelling, where he had scored in the eightieth percentile. Overall, his test scores were far below average.

Why had Westley's scores dropped? He'd been wearing a cast while he was taking the test, and I wondered whether it had distracted him. Weeks before, he had hurt himself during a game of hide-and-seek. Erik had also injured himself during the game—the boys had managed to fall out a window. My father, who had dropped by for a visit, went into Westley and Erik's bedroom to find the boys; he didn't see them behind the window curtain, where they were hiding. Taking a break from hide-and-seek, my father sat down in the living room to talk to me. Suddenly, we heard crying and screaming in the backyard.

We were dumbfounded by how the boys had gotten there, given that there wasn't a door in the back of the house, until we realized that their weight had pushed out the window screen, causing them to fall backward out the window. Fortunately, we lived in a one-story house. Nonetheless, Erik had fractured his left arm and elbow, while Westley had fractured his left wrist. Their injuries made the boys the talk of the school. When I took them to their classrooms after they had their casts put on, it was priceless to see the reactions and double takes of the other students. It was, of course, far less amusing to later see Westley's test scores. I had hoped the cast was to blame.

Fifth Grade

As my boys entered the fifth grade, I was already thinking ahead to another milestone; I couldn't believe that my boys would start middle school in one year. I was determined to make this fifth grade really count to get the boys on track.

School had only been in session for a week when I went to New York for my sister's wedding. I was gone five days. My husband brought the kids with him to pick me up at the airport. I hardly recognized Westley. He had severe facial tics, and his face was in spasm. I had never witnessed anything like it. Chris and I knew that it was probably stress; Westley had just started a new school year, and I had been away from him only once before, several years ago. Fortunately, the tics subsided over the next few days.

Westley's handwriting remained illegible most of the time. His fifth-grade teacher was very patient with him. She said that when he slowed down and made an effort, he could produce excellent work. He continued to be a great writer with many creative ideas. But his teacher was still concerned about his organization skills and neatness, especially in math operations, such as division and fractions.

Erik had many friends and loved school. In spite of his hyperactivity and distractibility, he was succeeding in the classroom. His teacher had a great sense of humor, which kept his interest. He continued to excel in history and did well in all other subjects. It seemed that my husband had been right about Ritalin. There was not enough of a problem to warrant it, though Erik's motor mouth was still very much present.

Westley was beginning to make new friends. But he still was overly eager to please his peers, which made him an easy target for some of the meaner kids. They would dare him to do silly things, and in an attempt to fit in, he would do them. When the recess bell rang, the children were to walk to get in line with their class-mates. Kids would dare Westley to run and scream while going to the class line. And he'd do it, even as the other students laughed at him. On top of that, Erik would tell me that his brother frequently talked to himself at school, and some kids couldn't resist teasing him.

One boy was a bit more mature than the rest. He would tell Westley that he had a choice, that he did not have to listen to those kids. He turned out to be Westley's best friend that year.

Westley still remained irritable at home, and we were constantly breaking up fights between him and Erik. Erik would tease Westley, and then Westley would physically attack him. Sometimes, if Erik just looked at him with an odd expression, Westley would fly off the handle. He never seemed happy. Going out to dinner or on vacations would often turn into a disaster. There was always a dark cloud around him. My husband and I were becoming very concerned because Westley was now physically strong and capable of causing serious injury to his brother. We hesitated to seek therap—we didn't want to hear the Ritalin rap again.

A well-known homeopathic (natural medicine) practitioner in Santa Monica—Murray Clarke—was recommended to me. Many parents had turned to him while seeking alternative ways to address their children's ADHD diagnosis.

Dr. Clarke observed Westley and Erik, and took a hair analysis to check for toxic elements and heavy metal poisoning. He ordered blood work to test for food allergies and examine their general blood chemistry. The results of the hair anal-ysis showed a high level of lead, especially with Erik. Their general blood chemistry was within normal range. The food allergy test for Westley indicated a peanut allergy. Erik's test showed he had an allergy to peanuts, gluten, and garlic. Unfortunately, we couldn't continue to take the kids to the homoeopathic doc-tor—our insurance wouldn't cover it.

I showed their pediatrician the test results. He didn't give much weight to the hair analysis, but he did order a finger-prick blood test to check lead levels. Normal levels fall between one to nine micrograms per deciliter (mcg/dl). Westley's test showed four mcg/dl. Erik's test came back with a result of eight mcg/dl, a little on the high side but still in the normal range. The doctor wanted to recheck Erik's lead level in a few months.

I told my own doctor about the results, and he suggested that I give Erik 2,000 milligrams of vitamin C a day to help remove the lead from his system (a pro-cess called detoxification). His lead level was checked two months later; it had dropped from eight mcg/dl to two mcg/dl.

Although the boys' lead levels fell within the normal range, there may be reason to doubt that "normal" and "healthy" are the same thing. An episode of the acclaimed PBS series *Now,* hosted by Bill Moyers, cited studies indicating that lead levels as low as three mcg/dl can impair a child's health. Another study, published in the *New England Journal of Medicine,* found that even lead levels below the federal and international guidelines of ten micrograms per deciliter produce a large drop in IQ—up to 7.4 points. Disturbingly, researchers estimate that one out of every ten U.S. children has levels of five mcg/dl or above.

Having addressed the boys' lead levels, I wanted to seek solutions to their other problems, too. Because of his allergy, I tried to get Erik off wheat products; it was impossible. He complained that it was bad enough I had taken dairy away from him. His health was good, and he had an excellent school attendance record, so I let it slide.

Meanwhile, Westley continued to exhibit facial tics, and I wanted to seek medical help for him. I took him to a neurologist. His symptoms were mild; she didn't observe any neurological problems and agreed the tics were stress related. I noticed that when he had problems with the kids at school, the severity of his facial tics would increase. He would do anything to make friends. He was easily led and quite naïve. Westley would get into more trouble than the kids who were daring him. He could not comprehend that the children were laughing at him and that they weren't really his friends. His behavior was becoming even more eccentric, and he didn't fit in with the other kids. When Westley did make a friend, the other kids would tease the student, and that would put an end to it. I couldn't even begin to imagine what it was going to be like in middle school for him.

Away from school, he would attack Erik over little things. Westley had a sweet side, but he often gave in to rage. He had absolutely no impulse control. Erik was beginning to fear him.

I had yet another reason to worry: Westley was shutting me out. He used to share his feelings with me; now he would tell me that he was fine even though it was obvious he was not. I told him that I loved him unconditionally and that he could tell me anything. I was there to help. He needed an ally more than ever.

Westley was becoming more withdrawn and had a new obsession: *Dragon Ball Z.* He drew hundreds of sketches of the cartoon characters. The drawings were quite good, considering how terrible his handwriting was. He played with the *Dragon Ball Z* figures and chewed on the tops of their heads. When I took the figures away from him, he would throw a tantrum and promise not to chew on them. But without even realizing it, he would put toys right back in his mouth.

Both my husband and I were very baffled as to why Westley was so angry. We were aware that he might be jealous of his brother, but he had everything a child could need. We were a loving and supportive family. I was thinking it was possible that his irritability came from spending the first months of his life so ill. Being on a ventilator and being gavage-fed may have had some deep, negative psychological impact on him. Perhaps there was something wrong with the wiring in his brain from being born so prematurely. We had no choice but to look into family counseling. Hoping that a psychotherapist would know how to reach him, we began family counseling at Vista Del Mar Child and Family Services. The boys enjoyed the sessions. They both expressed their feelings well, but Westley continued to exhibit an angry attitude, while Erik was always fidgety.

Fifth grade flew by so fast. Having their elementary school right behind our house had been a great experience, and I was a bit overwhelmed by the thought of the boys going to middle school, where there were more than 1,800 students. Westley was still weak in areas of organization and neatness. I was also concerned for him socially. I know how awfully mean middle school kids can be. According to his teacher, he had made good academic progress, although his Stanford 9 scores did not reflect his teacher's findings. His spelling score remained very high, in the eighty-first percentile. The total reading score was very poor, in the twenty-fourth percentile. His math scores were in the twenty-first percentile, and his total language score had bottomed out in the ninth percentile.

The summer going into sixth grade was a busy one. We were moving again, and we continued family therapy. At the end of the family counseling session, the psychotherapist asked me in private if I had ever heard of Asperger's syndrome. She described it as a high-functioning type of autism, suggested that Westley be evaluated for it, and recommended that I read *Asperger's Syndrome: A Guide for Parents and Professionals* by Tony Attwood (Jessica Kingsley Publishers, 1998).

After reading the book, I thought there was a strong possibility that Westley did have Asperger's syndrome, even though he did not exhibit all the symptoms. He didn't lack empathy, which is one of the characteristics of Asperger's, but he was quite naïve and had little ability to form friendships. At times he exhibited repetitive speech and obsessed on his latest fixation. He was very clumsy and had odd postures, all symptoms of Asperger's. I took him to be evaluated by a licensed clinical psychologist, and her diagnostic impressions were as follows:

1. Asperger's syndrome
2. Expressive language disorder
3. Phonological disorder
4. Learning disorder, not otherwise specified

After receiving the report, I spoke with the psychologist. She told me that while Westley exhibited Asperger-like symptoms, he had more of a social learning disability; unlike Asperger's sufferers, Westley did desire emotional connection. No matter what the official diagnosis was, I was very concerned that Westley was entering middle school with very little educational support. Being his mother, I could not help feeling a great deal of guilt. I blamed myself for letting him fall through the cracks. I would have to act quickly to get the services he needed.

Sixth Grade

Both Chris and I knew that Westley was going to need help and possibly be medicated for his anger. I had him assessed by a psychiatrist to consider a medicine trial. Her diagnosis included ADHD, Asperger's syndrome, and oppositional disorder. She was reluctant to prescribe Ritalin because of his facial tics, which were quite apparent in our sessions with her. After researching all the different medicines, we decided to try a drug called Risperdal (generically known as risperidone). It would address both his attention disorder and irritability, and it was not a stimulant.

As soon as school started, I requested an emergency Individualized Education Program meeting. The guidance counselor was helpful and set up an academic performance test. Westley's math scores were very weak, and he qualified for a math resource at school.

The Individualized Education Program meeting was held in November. It was decided that Westley would continue with adaptive physical education and a weekly full-inclusion teacher would visit his classroom to assist his other teachers. His handwriting was so poor that we requested he receive an AlphaSmart keyboard to type all his work. The school said he no longer qualified for speech therapy, although he could not be understood a quarter of the time. The public school system could only do so much to address his needs.

Erik sailed beautifully into middle school. He was receiving all As and Bs except for math, where he was getting Cs. His English teacher recommended him for the leadership program. He declined because he wanted to stay in chorus and he couldn't do both. He was making new friends. The only challenge that remained was getting him to do his homework.

Westley was receiving mostly Cs in his classes. No one could read his handwriting, and the AlphaSmart keyboard never arrived as promised. Westley made a few friends in his adaptive P.E. class. He was a little upset and self-conscious because some children in the class were quite mentally handicapped. I told him that he could go into regular P.E. but also explained that it was very competitive. He decided to stay in adaptive P.E.

Some of the kids at school continued to make fun of Westley and dare him to do inappropriate things. One boy dared him to call his math teacher a bitch, and he did and received detention. He wrote his teacher a heartfelt apology letter, saying that he knew what he said was not true and he was very sorry. He blamed no one but himself.

The Risperdal did seem to take the edge off his anger. The boys would still fight, but not as often. The most negative side effect was that the medicine made Westley tired. He had a difficult time waking up in the morning even though he had enough sleep. We knew that the Risperdal was only going to be a temporary solution.

Still researching natural health and alternative medicine, I began to suspect that Westley might have candidiasis—an overgrowth of a common yeast in the

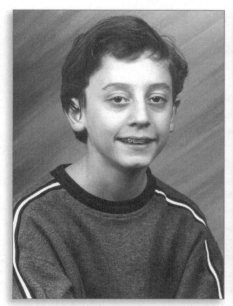 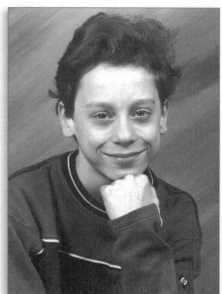

Erik and Westley in sixth grade

intestines. Symptoms of yeast-connected problems are fatigue, irritability, short attention span, headaches, and respiratory problems, just to name a few. One of the causes of this condition is the overuse of antibiotics. His medical file showed he had experienced thirty-five rounds of antibiotics before he was six years old. He was still taking antibiotics frequently for his countless sinus infections.

My children's pediatrician was not knowledgeable about alternative medicine, so I asked my own doctor to order a candidiasis test for Westley. The test results came back showing that he was abnormally high in all three categories he was tested for, including IgG (long-term blood infection), IgM (acute infection), and IgA (infection in the gastrointestinal tract and the bowels). My doctor prescribed nystatin, an antifungal medicine.

In addition to antibiotics, sugar can also cause an overgrowth of yeast in the intestines. I made an effort to feed my kids organic fruit after school instead of sweets. We would allow them to have soda when we went out to dinner, a once-a-week occurrence.

One of these restaurant excursions resulted in an eye-opening experience. Westley had spaghetti and a soft drink for dinner. He began to act silly and had his knife on his lap. I asked him to put the knife on his plate. He did, then smiled, and put his fork on his lap. I wasn't amused—and became even less so when he used my sleeve to wipe his face. I realized at this point that he was intoxicated on wheat and sugar. My husband had been in the restroom while this behavior was going on. Westley managed to pull himself together as his father dragged him out of the restaurant.

Often, the connection between the boys' behavior and what they ate was read-ily apparent. I avoided taking them to the supermarket, where they would beg me to buy junk food—exactly the type of food that could have the most nightmar-ish effect on their behavior. When they were eleven, Erik talked me into buying a multicolored fruit-flavor bar. At home, after eating only half their treats, both boys became hyperactive and out of control. I was confronted with two "Tasmanian devils," and it was obvious to me that their behavior was connected to what they had just eaten. I threw the rest of the bars away after looking at the nutritional information on the box. The ingredients were water, sugar, corn syrup, high fruc-tose corn syrup, natural and artificial flavoring, citric acid, guar gum, locust bean, Red No. 40, Blue No. 1, and Yellow Nos. 5 and 6. I have since learned that arti-ficial food colorings have been linked to allergies, asthma, and hyperactivity; they are also a possible carcinogen.

Sixth grade was over, and Westley had straight Cs, except for a D in math and an A in his keyboard class. The Stanford 9 results were encouraging. Westley's math score was in the fortieth percentile—quite an improvement from the year before, when his scores hit the twenty-first percentile. His reading score also increased, from the twenty-fourth percentile to the thirty-third. The greatest improvement was in his language skills, which had ranked in the ninth percentile in fifth grade and were now the fortieth percentile. He scored in the fifty-second percentile in lan-guage mechanics. I was relieved.

Erik's Stanford 9 results were all above average except for his spelling and math scores, which ranked in the twenty-second and thirty-eighth percentile, respectively.

The psychotherapist recommended that I enroll Westley in a social skills group with psychologist Carol Hirschfield. She had developed the group for children who faced challenges like Westley's. The psychotherapist suggested that it would help Westley improve his relations with his peers. I enrolled both of the boys. Erik loved it; Westley hated it. He would rather be home playing computer games or watching his favorite TV show, *Seventh Heaven*. I begged him to give the social skills group a chance, and I told him that if after one month he was still unhap-py, he could stop going.

We decided to take Westley off the Risperdal. He was just too tired every morning, even though he was on a very low dosage. He was still exhibiting facial tics. My commitment to exploring alternative medicine was stronger than ever, and I knew there had to be something more natural that could help him without negative side effects.

Seventh Grade: Finding Answers

The boys continued with their weekly social skills group after school start-ed. Westley would protest as we drove to the sessions, and he would argue with Erik on the way to the group and on the way home. I knew it was going to take a lot of persuading to make him keep going. So I decided that if the kids earned enough points, they would be able to pick out a toy at the end of the session. Unfortunately, Westley never earned enough points, which agitated him that much more. Even so, the group provided a safe environment for the kids to express themselves and discuss their everyday problems.

Erik's ongoing chattering remained one of his biggest challenges. He had a loud voice, and I could hear him talking while I sat in the waiting room. Once, I heard him complaining about me. He was angry at how fanatical I had become about his diet and vitamin supplements. He was sick of it and said it was not helping because he was still too skinny.

One afternoon I had Erik join me while I walked the dog. He spent the whole time telling me off. All his friends ate junk food and dairy products, he said, and they were healthy. He was embarrassed by how strict I was and was going to eat whatever he wanted from now on, including hot dogs (which are loaded with nitrates, known to cause behavior problems). Erik ended the conversation by telling me that other than the "diet stuff," he still liked me. He was making me laugh and cry at the same time.

Westley was falling flat on his face in seventh grade. His handwriting looked like scribbling. He would start writing in the middle of the page, and the words would run together. It was impossible to read what he wrote. The full-inclusion teacher repeatedly told me she was working to get him an AlphaSmart keyboard. Westley began to give up. He would rather not try at all than to try and fail. His teacher said he was missing assignments and that the work he turned in wasn't acceptable.

There was always a lot of pressure connected with getting the boys ready for school. Erik would sneak away from his breakfast to watch cartoons. He would wait to the very last second to get dressed. One morning both children were running very late, and I heard a commotion upstairs. The boys were fighting, and I broke them up and hurried them out the front door so they wouldn't miss their ride to school. I picked them up after school, and Erik came out first. There were severe red scratches all across his face. "What did you tell your friends about your face?" I asked him. He said he had told them he had fallen and scratched himself. Then Westley came out, looking no better than his brother. "What did you tell your friends?" I asked. His answer had been more straightforward—he had told them that he had gotten into a cat fight with his brother.

The boys were not getting along at all, and Erik was becoming more aggressive out of self-defense. I was at a loss and didn't know what to do next. I hoped that the social skills group would be able to help them work it out.

Erik was becoming more hyperactive. He would walk across the back of the couch or climb all over it as he watched television; the cushions would be thrown all over the room. At times he was not as hyper, and I realized that when he was on antibiotics—particularly Zithromax (azithromycin)—his hyperactivity increased.

Westley's test scores were still very poor, mostly because of his handwriting. His science teacher gave him a zero on a test and, next to the grade, wrote, "I can't read this paper." Westley had been promised an AlphaSmart keyboard one year before. It finally arrived, but it was defective and could not print out his work. It was November, and nothing was going right for him. He received an F on a history test. His teacher gave him a chance to retake the exam, but he didn't bother to study for it. He didn't seem to care anymore. His backpack was always filled with crinkled paper, bulging out of his folders. The only good news was that Westley wasn't getting as many respiratory infections as before. I thought that possibly the nystatin treatment for his candidiasis was improving his health.

Other than the first several months after my children's birth, I was experiencing the darkest moments of my motherhood. I was confused and clueless as to what to do next to help Westley. I felt it was a hopeless situation. I had tried everything and at this point had to let go and put it into God's hands. After my kids left for school I sat down and prayed, fervently. My prayer was soon to be answered in a big way.

Feeling fatigued, anxious, and depressed, I went to see David Allen, MD, for an acupuncture treatment. He was already well aware of the situation with my children, and I told him how Westley's constant irritability and violent temper seemed to be getting worse. In response, Dr. Allen suggested that Westley undergo quantitative electroencephalography (QEEG), a "brain mapping" procedure, to determine whether seizures were behind his behavior. We scheduled an appointment.

In the meantime, Westley's psychologist called me and told me that there was no way that the Los Angeles Unified School District (LAUSD) could meet all of his needs. She told me about a private school called Village Glen. They had recently opened a campus not too far from our neighborhood. The school served children with social and communication disabilities, including high-functioning autism and Asperger's. Social skills and expressive language were emphasized in every class. I visited the campus the following week, and I was impressed with the program as well as the staff. The school's capacity was two hundred students, but at the time there were only seventy-one students enrolled.

I contacted the Regional Center to have Westley evaluated one more time for Asperger's and for educational support. The same doctor did the evaluation and said that Westley did not have Asperger's. Her diagnostic impressions were as follows:

1. Highly scattered cognitive abilities

2. Unclear articulation to the degree he is quite difficult to understand at least twenty-five percent of the time

3. Poor perception of body and space

4. History of facial tics; some periods of shuddering were observed

5. Impulsivity; social immaturity

At the follow-up with the doctor, she asked me whether anyone had ever diagnosed Westley as having cerebral palsy. She said it could be connected to the neonatal risk factors, which probably contributed to his articulation difficulties, gross motor awkwardness, and fine motor challenges. I told her that a pediatrician had ruled out cerebral palsy when he was two and a half years old because he had been walking in an age-appropriate manner. She then wondered whether his disabilities might have come from organic impairment, a result of the premature birth. Because Westley was very engaging during the assessment, she said the diagnosis of Asperger's was no longer appropriate. Regardless, we all believed that he would benefit from a school such as Village Glen to meet his needs with his expressive language delays and social learning disability.

Westley's psychologist attended the Individualized Education Program meeting to support us in getting the approval we needed from the school administration to let Westley go to Village Glen. All of his academic teachers reported that he had a great deal of difficulty paying attention and staying on task. He would become confused and forget what he was supposed to do on his assignments. He often would not be able to find his work in his messy backpack. He constantly needed one-on-one assistance from the teachers. He had a great deal of difficulty with visual-motor integration and auditory processing, which affected his ability to write notes, copy information, and express his thoughts in writing.

The occupational assessment reported that Westley's hand manipulation skills were in decline, as was his visual-motor control when performing handwriting activities; he could not read his own handwriting. He had trouble focusing on important points and tended to get hung up on irrelevant details. All the teachers were going out of their way to accommodate him in the class by photocopying other students' notes and giving him more time to complete the assignments. According to all his teachers, his main problem was missing work.

We also feared for Westley's safety. He had many challenges with impulse control, and the middle school kids were always trying to make him say and do mean things to the other students. If a child told him to kick someone, he would. He had difficulty understanding social nuances. He just wanted to make friends and to be accepted by his peers. For safety's sake, we had to get him out of public middle school.

All the school staff members unanimously agreed that Los Angeles Unified School District should let Westley attend a nonpublic school and that LAUSD should pay for it. We were very relieved; unfortunately, Westley was not crazy about the idea of leaving his few friends.

With all the problems in his current school, he still resisted going to Village Glen. There were two more weeks of class before winter break. He wanted to go back to his public school after winter break for three more weeks and finish out the semester. We allowed him to do so, and I assured him that if he was unhappy with Village Glen, he could always return to a public school.

Some of my siblings and good friends were worried about Westley's lack of progress. They said I had waited long enough, and out of concern for him, they advised me to try a trial run of Ritalin. I thanked everyone for their input and told them about the imminent QEEG brain map, which, we hoped, would offer some answers.

0011 Amino Acid Analysis - 20 Plasma		Methodology: ION Exchange HPLC

Essential Amino Acids	Results	Reference Limits (For adults 13 and over)	Low Limit	High Limit
Arginine	90	70 - 160	70	160
Histidine	71	65 - 150	65	150
Isoleucine	51	50 - 160	50	160
Leucine	102 L	105 - 250	105	250
Lysine	138 L	140 - 250	140	250
Methionine	24	20 - 60	20	60
Phenylalanine	46	45 - 140	45	140
Threonine	109	85 - 250	85	250
Tryptophan	55	45 - 120	45	120
Valine	174 L	180 - 480	180	480

umo/L

Essential Amino Acid Derivatives

Neuroendocrine Metabolism	Results	Reference Limits	Low Limit	High Limit
Glycine	209	200 - 450	200	450
Serine	77 L	80 - 200	80	200
Taurine	50	50 - 250	50	250
Tyrosine	61	50 - 120	50	120

Ammonia/Energy Metabolism	Results	Reference Limits	Low Limit	High Limit
Asparagine	37	35 - 100	35	100
Aspartic Acid	9	6 - 30	6	30
Citruline	38	15 - 70	15	70
Glutamic Acid	53	45 - 200	45	200
Glutamine	572	500 - 1,050	500	1050
Ornithine	82	35 - 100	35	100

Westley's amino acid profile

The day of Westley's appointment arrived. To begin the procedure, a technician pasted sensors on Westley's head that would record his brainwaves as he performed math problems, reading, and other tasks. The machine also recorded his brainwaves as he shut his eyes and relaxed. One and a half hours later, the procedure was complete.

My husband and I went to Dr. Allen's office to get the test results. The QEEG report showed abnormal activity in Westley's brain. Frankly, we weren't surprised. His brain had a marked excess of episodic anterior high-voltage fast activity, as well as episodes of frontal dominant slow (theta) activity. In lay terms, parts of his brain were moving too slowly, while other parts were moving too fast. The doctor described it as playing a football game with all of the players running at different speeds. His brain was missing the relaxation type of rhythm, which created seizure-like activity in his brain. This discovery would explain why Westley was irritable so much of the time. He had a hyperreactive brain with little threshold. According to our doctor, if

0011 Amino Acid Analysis - 20 Plasma			Methodology: ION Exchange HPLC	
Essential Amino Acids	Results	Reference Limits (For adults 13 and over)	Low Limit	High Limit
Arginine	84	70 - 160	70	160
Histidine	68	65 - 150	65	150
Isoleucine	49 L	50 - 160	50	160
Leucine	102 L	105 - 250	105	250
Lysine	133 L	140 - 250	140	250
Methionine	23	20 - 60	20	60
Phenylalanine	45	45 - 140	45	140
Threonine	84 L	85 - 250	85	250
Tryptophan	45	45 - 120	45	120
Valine	190	180 - 480	180	480
Essential Amino Acid Derivatives				umo/L
Neuroendocrine Metabolism			Low Limit	High Limit
Glycine	228	200 - 450	200	450
Serine	97	80 - 200	80	200
Taurine	31 L	50 - 250	50	250
Tyrosine	61	50 - 120	50	120
Ammonia/Energy Metabolism			Low Limit	High Limit
Asparagine	36	35 - 100	35	100
Aspartic Acid	7	6 - 30	6	30
Citruline	22	15 - 70	15	70
Glutamic Acid	51	45 - 200	45	200
Glutamine	491 L	500 - 1,050	500	1050
Ornithine	54	35 - 100	35	100

Erik's amino acid profile

we had put him on Ritalin or any other stimulant, it would have most likely made him worse or even had caused him to have a convulsion, one of the many side effects of the drug.

My husband's hunches were correct all along about not medicating Westley. Usually the antiseizure medicine Depakote (generically known as divalproex sodium) would be recommended for Westley's type of brain activity. Depakote has many side effects, and our doctor said Westley should first undergo an amino acid panel test. Low amino acid levels could be contributing to his abnormal brain activity.

Chris took Westley in for the test the day after Christmas. In Westley's usual manner he created quite a scene at the doctor's office, throwing a tantrum as the nurse drew his blood.

Three agonizing weeks later, we received the test results. The test measures levels of twenty amino acids. Westley had four in the low range and sixteen in the medium-low range—a significant amino acid deficiency.

Either Westley was not getting enough protein in his diet or he had poor digestive absorption. Dr. Allen prescribed four free-form amino acid capsules, to be taken on an empty stomach two times a day. He also prescribed additional amino acid supplements, including one taurine tablet, one GABA (gamma-aminobutyric acid) tablet, and two inositol tablets, to be taken with breakfast and dinner. Vitamin B_6 was prescribed to help with the metabolism of the amino acids, and Dr. Allen suggested a multivitamin and cod liver oil (an essential fatty acid source) to help support the neurological connections in Westley's brain. The doctor said that we should start seeing an improvement within a few weeks.

I went home and read everything I could find in my nutrition books about amino acids. Westley was low in the amino acid lysine; low lysine levels could cause low energy, inability to concentrate, and irritability. Westley's taurine levels were also extremely low, a deficiency that could lead to tics, epilepsy, anxiety, hyperactivity, and poor brain function. Some of Westley's most significant challenges were symptoms of low amino acid levels.

Even so, I did not have any great expectations for a positive outcome. The other measures we had tried had helped somewhat—we'd removed dairy from his diet, addressed his candidiasis with nystatin, and turned to Risperdal for his attention disorder and anger. Unfortunately, nothing to this point had made a big difference in his violent behavior, poor impulse control, impaired attention, or facial tics.

Yet after Westley's first week of taking the amino acid supplements, I noticed that there had been no bickering between the kids. This change was a miracle in itself. Moreover, Westley was going out of his way to talk to me after years of being distant and cranky. His psychologist commented on how much more Westley was participating in the social-skills group. The cloud was lifting from him. I was no longer observing facial tics or twitches. I knew that the amino acids were working.

Westley attended his new school in the beginning of February. The bus picked him up and dropped him off at our home. On the first day of school he was nervous, but he handled the transition very well. His class had nine students, one teacher, and an aide. The students welcomed him, and he made new friends in no time. He was where he was supposed to be.

After three weeks at his new school, he came home one afternoon, and when I opened the door, there stood Westley with a happy grin from ear to ear. He could not stop smiling. His voice brimming with emotion, he announced, "I love life!"

The amino acids were the missing link. He continued to improve in his school performance. His grades went from Cs and Ds to As and Bs. He was doing his homework independently. One Sunday, when he went up to his room for a couple of hours, I assumed he was playing computer games. Instead, he was typing his book report on his computer and printing it out without anyone's assistance. He received an A- on his report. We were very proud of him.

Because an apple does not fall far from the tree, I thought it would be a good idea to have my and Erik's amino acid levels checked. I was shocked when the results came back. Our amino acid levels were lower than Westley's! I was not as surprised about Erik, because he is the pickier eater of the two. He had never cared for protein foods, such as poultry, fish, beef, beans, and nuts. Erik was at the bottom of the low on tryptophan. Tryptophan is a precursor to serotonin and helps control hyperactivity in children. Erik had always been the more hyper one. He began taking a tryptophan supplement before bed and, after a week, calmed down substantially.

My own test results were alarming. Out of the twenty amino acids tested, thirteen were low. The remaining seven were in the medium-low range. I had a low-protein diet. With my stressful life, the little protein that I was consuming would be immediately zapped up. I ordered a custom-made amino acid compound. Dr. Allen also prescribed tyrosine, phenylalanine, and glutamine. Within one week I felt an increase of energy and I was more alert. Life didn't seem like such a burden anymore. I was experiencing firsthand Westley's happy mood. I actually felt giddy. I had no idea how depressed I had been all that time. I had been so overly consumed with my kids' issues that I had no energy or time to take care of myself.

Eighth Grade

By this time, the boys had taken amino acid supplements for more than one and a half years. Westley continued to receive As and Bs on his report cards. At school, he was awarded Most Improved Student of the Year in behavior and social skills. Westley had not scratched, hit, kicked, or bitten his brother since the amino acid supplements were introduced, although Erik continued to

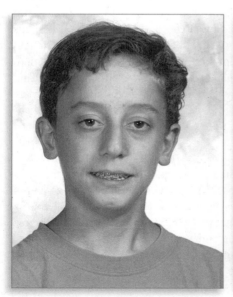 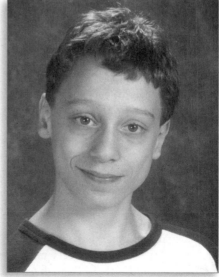

Erik and Westley in eighth grade

tease him relentlessly. This teasing upset Westley, but he expressed himself verbally instead of giving in to violent impulses. I no longer observed facial tics or twitches in Westley.

Erik received good grades in school until the seventh and eight grades. He scored well on tests, but getting him to do his homework was a constant challenge. Erik thought he spent enough time working at school, and he believed that after school was his own time to use as he pleased, which he did mostly by playing addictive computer games. His grades fluctuated between Bs and Ds.

Concerned by this change, I spoke with Erik's guidance counselor about his sudden decline in grades. She said this was typical of adolescent boys; once he got into high school, his grades should turn around. But Erik always said that his middle school experience trained him to hate going to school. He felt like a victim of a low-quality education, even though he did enjoy English and choir.

High School

Westley continued to study at Village Glen and felt comfortable there. Socially, Westley remained somewhat withdrawn. He had a few friends, but he didn't reach out to other students. Westley complained about classmates annoying or teasing him. Although he rarely raised his hand in class to answer questions, his teachers knew he paid good attention; he always had the correct answer when called upon. His teachers believed Westley was self-conscious due to his speech impediment. He excelled in English, but math was difficult for him. On the Wide Range Achievement Test, he scored at the high-school level in reading and spelling, but he scored a mere sixth-grade equivalency in math. He did poorly with standardized tests but passed his algebra quizzes in class. Perhaps Westley's biggest obstacle in math class was the other students' disruptive behaviors. He complained that his teachers spent more time disciplining than teaching.

During Westley's ninth grade Individualized Education Program, my husband and I were pleasantly surprised and awed by Westley's creative writing sample, where he scored above college level. He had never expressed himself verbally in the manner in which he wrote. Westley had shown great strength in creative writing since second grade. Both of my husband's parents were professional writers, and apparently Westley had inherited their writing genes.

Even though he never read his grandfather's work, Westley wrote in the same fashion. Milton Merlin was a studied philosopher and spent decades staying up until three or four in the morning reading, writing, and listening to classical music. Unfortunately, Milton passed away when the boys were seven years old. Even though we lived nearby, the boys didn't spend enough time with Milton; between his advance into extreme old age and my boys' struggle with ADHD, it was a poor match. Nevertheless, Westley was very much like Milton.

Mr. Pope, Westley's English teacher, stated on his report card that Westley's deep and insightful work was a joy to read and quite refreshing. Westley liked

Mr. Pope best among his teachers because of his affable, philosophical, complex nature and deep approach to classwork. Westley claimed that he had found philosophy intensely interesting ever since first grade but never had the opportunity to express it until Mr. Pope's class.

In ninth grade, Westley received straight Bs, with the exception of a C in Spanish. At the meeting for Westley's tenth grade Individualized Education Program, the school administrators recommended that Westley be mainstreamed for two classes at his home high school. But Westley refused, since it meant he would have to wake up earlier; at this point Westley's bedtime was 1:00 a.m.

Overall, Westley was well liked by his teachers, and he turned in all his assignments in on time, if not early. He improved academically each year. In twelfth grade, Westley received straight As in all of his classes and Es for excellent effort in work habits and cooperation. He continued to use his AlphaSmart keyboard to help him type assignments, since his handwriting remained impossible to read.

The budget cutbacks that limited high school physical education to two years were a huge misfortune for my boys. They were never self-starters when it came to exercise. Regular exercise was crucial for their mental as well as physical health and well-being. At Westley's school, the social skills class was considered an important component. Personally, I believe that team sports would have taught him social interaction more effectively than four years of repetitive role playing in a social skills class.

Erik caused me serious concern; his grades dropped badly in middle school, and his new high school had 3,400 students with overcrowded classrooms. Los Angeles schools have their share of gangs, and Erik's was no exception. Luckily, Erik was admitted into the Communications Arts Academy. This program had special funding, which allowed for smaller classes, and focused on exposing students to colleges specializing in fine and graphic arts, film, and journalism. To remain in the program, students had to maintain GPA, attendance, and behavior standards.

Erik's freshman year started out with Cs and Bs but dropped to four Ds and an F in his health class by the end. He attended summer school to improve his grades. In tenth grade Erik's grades improved somewhat, but he did receive a D in Spanish. Erik passed his tests, but missing assignments hurt his grades. Teachers commented on his report cards that he was a pleasure to have in the class but frequently failed to turn in homework. Erik was well liked by his teachers and his peers; he had a disarming personality and always treated people respectfully.

But Erik's extreme laziness and lack of motivation worried me. All of his free time was spent on the couch watching television or playing computer games. Fortunately, Erik enjoyed educational television like the Discovery and History channels. He'd watch the news every day while preparing for school, which kept him well informed. Erik's quick-witted humor kept me laughing even when I was upset with him. As Erik's guidance counselor predicted, his grades did improve, but not until his junior year. He was finally doing his homework, but not until the morning it was due. I found it interesting that he received mostly As and a few Bs in English and History honor classes.

Miraculously, Erik returned from the living dead during his senior year. He took an after-school film appreciation class in the fall semester, and joined the after-school swimming team in the spring semester. Erik discovered his passion for filmmaking. His film teacher introduced him to a summer school program called Inner City Filmmakers (ICF). The program was started after the Rodney King riots with the intention of teaching at-risk youth how to make films. Students learned the process of writing a script, casting a project, shooting, editing, and overall production.

After graduation, Erik was accepted into ICF. It was an intense summer program during which the students often worked twelve hours a day. This experience matured Erik. He learned responsibility and organization.

Deepak Chopra says that instead of tutoring children in subjects in which they experience difficulty, it would be far wiser to tutor them in the area where they're gifted; make the most of the areas where children are gifted, instead of forcing them to learn something that doesn't come naturally. For Erik and Westley, adopting this approach made all the difference between their success and failure.

College

Erik and Westley recently finished their first year at Santa Monica City College. Westley is majoring in computer science, and Erik is majoring in film. They're both attending college full-time.

Over the past year, Erik completed an internship at Sony Pictures Entertainment. In addition to college, Erik is also working thirty hours a week at a movie theater, saving for his first car.

The California Department of Rehabilitation is helping Westley find employment; his fine motor skills remain a continuing challenge and struggle.

In addition to taking nutritional supplements, my children continue to eat healthfully, avoiding the foods that exacerbated their worst behaviors. It was no easy task to make dietary changes with my children; they're stubborn and picky eaters. I took them to natural food markets and allowed them to explore. Most delicatessens provide free samples, which gave them an opportunity to try out new foods. I ultimately succeeded in changing the way my children eat because I made them a part of the process. They remain in excellent health with a solid school attendance record.

Looking Back

I initially thought all of my children's health issues and developmental delays were a result of their premature birth. Although premature infants are at risk for developmental delays, I now believe there were other contributing factors—such as vaccines.

Why? The measles-mump-rubella vaccine is highly immunogenic, meaning it stimulates the immune system. Many children with ADHD, learning disabilities, and developmental delays also have autoimmune dysfunction, with several allergies to foods, drugs, and environmental toxins.

Numerous newspaper and magazine articles have questioned whether mercury in the environment and childhood vaccines (all contained mercury prior to 1999, and some still do) could be connected to autism and attention disorders. Mercury and aluminum toxicity has also been linked to arthritis, asthma, allergies, Alzheimer's, diabetes, multiple sclerosis, fibromyalgia, lupus, chronic fatigue syndrome, depression, bipolar disorder, schizophrenia, seizures, and learning disabilities.

In their book *A Shot in the Dark* (Avery Publishing, 1991), authors Harris L. Coulter and Barbara Loe Fisher list the following conditions that indicate when a vaccine should be withheld:

- A history of seizures or other neurological diseases in the child or other member of the immediate family
- A history of allergy to components used in the vaccines, such as eggs, gelatin, casein, or thimerosal (which contains mercury)
- Premature birth or low birth weight
- A chronic or recent illness
- A parent or sibling with a vaccine reaction
- A prior severe reaction to a vaccination

If I had known then what I know now, I would not have had my sons vaccinated; they had been born prematurely, their birth weights were low, and Westley had hyaline membrane disease. They both have asthma, symptoms of ADHD, and allergies to many foods, medicines, and environmental toxins. I can't help but wonder whether vaccinating my children contributed to many of these problems, including Westley's seizures. Heavy-metal tests in both of my children indicated aluminum and mercury were present, though not in the very elevated range. Regardless, there is no safe level for any heavy metal. Fortunately, supplementing Erik's and Westley's diets with amino acids and vitamin C helped lower their levels of toxic heavy metals.

I was unknowingly contributing to their symptoms by feeding them toxic foods, like cereals soaked with processed sugar and food dyes, ice cream, and other foods with artificial food coloring. I was clueless about the fact that most artificial coloring contains mercury, lead, and arsenic.

When I sought help for my kids' issues, Ritalin was always cast as the solution—the only solution. The doctors would evaluate Erik and Westley for twenty minutes and tell us that they needed to go on Ritalin. Not one of the psychiatrists, psychologists, or medical doctors ever addressed their diets or other possible causes. When I would ask them whether the boys' diets could be causing their symptoms, the reply would be that diet had nothing to do with it, and the cause was probably a chemical imbalance in the brain.

Westley's symptoms worsened as he got older. It was frightening to imagine where he could have wound up in life—he had been failing in school and was being easily led by the wrong kids. His violent temper and poor impulse control had been a great challenge for him. His facial tics were always present. I feared for him. What would have happened had he not undergone a QEEG or an amino acid test? Would he have run into trouble with the law? Would he have ultimately ended up in jail?

My most important lesson was learning to trust my instincts. I almost fell into the Ritalin trap, which would have harmed my boys, not healed them. Parents often know instinctively what's best for their children, but they need to learn to listen to their hearts instead of being blindly led by the pharmaceutical industry.

Alternative medicine and the heroic health care professionals who practice it saved my children, and I am deeply grateful.

TWO

From Sickness to Health

MY OWN JOURNEY

As I noted earlier, the apple doesn't fall far from the tree. Like my children, I have had the symptoms of an attention disorder my whole life. But I never had a label for my problems—until I learned about my kids' disorder.

Much of my life was spent struggling against attention problems—in addition to other health challenges, including frequent infections. In trying to get healthy, I saw doctor after doctor and ingested a pharmacological cornucopia of medicines, without any luck.

It was only after turning to natural medicine solutions and natural living that I began to transform my health. Today, after many years of suffering, I am finally strong, healthy, and happy.

A Lifetime of Illness

I remember how hard it was to pay attention in school. My greatest fear was that I wouldn't pass to the next grade level. Teachers frequently caught me daydreaming. In elementary school, although I did well on spelling tests and loved drawing, I was a slow reader, and math was challenging. I was also uncoordinated; in P.E., I was often the last kid picked to play on a team. I had a speech impediment, which the other kids teased me about, I was immature for my age, and my friendships never lasted long. I became a loner and suffered from low self-esteem.

To make matters worse, I was in a prestigious public school system in Ridgewood, New Jersey. Passing eighth grade became an uphill battle. Then, new problems emerged, compounding my academic difficulties. I started to experience regular respiratory infections, and teachers often told me that I looked tired.

By ninth grade, my family had moved to a new school district, and I was bringing my grades up (except in algebra, which I never passed). But my health problems persisted. My senior year, I began feeling weak and had low energy. My doctor ordered a general blood chemical panel. The test results indicated low thyroidal activity. Though a CAT scan was ordered, I never saw the results—the hospital lost my records, and I moved away to college without seeking additional medical attention for my thyroid.

In my early twenties, I was being treated for bronchitis when my doctor noticed a large goiter in my neck. A CAT scan indicated that I had hypothyroidism—an underactive thyroid. I was prescribed Synthroid (levothyroxine sodium), which I took until I was thirty years old. A doctor took me off the medicine to retest my thyroid; the test results showed it to be functioning within normal ranges.

Other than having an occasional respiratory infection and still experiencing the challenges of an undiagnosed attention disorder, my health was stable for several years—until my children began preschool. My immune system took hit after hit. I was catching all of their infections; I had frequent ear infections and chronic bronchitis. The medicines I was prescribed created new problems. Every time I took penicillin, bumps appeared on my fingers. My doctor switched me to the combination antibiotic Bactrim (sulfamethoxazole and trimethoprim). It didn't take much time for hives to appear on my arms. I was prescribed other antibiotics but had to go off them after a few days because of negative side effects.

Meanwhile, as doctors were recommending Ritalin for my children, I began wondering about my own attention disorder. Although my husband was opposed to Ritalin for Erik and Westley, I wanted to try it myself to see if it would alleviate my own behavioral challenges. After a psychiatric examination, I was prescribed Ritalin. But it was difficult to determine whether it was helping—I was chronically sick with ear infections, bronchitis, and chronic fatigue.

That's when the behavior specialist I was seeing for Westley and Erik suggested that I try an antidepressant. She said it would help take the edge off the stress of raising ADHD-diagnosed twins. I stopped Ritalin and was prescribed Zoloft. Within three days of taking the drug, my sex drive disappeared. My emotions felt as though they were trapped in a cave inside my brain. I was numb. The medicine actually made me depressed. I stopped Zoloft after a month. Soon afterward, I was diagnosed with Hashimoto's thyroiditis, an underactive thyroid disorder. I began taking Synthroid again.

At the same time, my ear infections were so persistent that I was experiencing vertigo. (One night, I became so dizzy that I couldn't walk two feet without losing my balance. I was worried; I had completed a course of antibiotics, and I still felt sick.) I often heard a loud ringing in my ears, and my brain felt fuzzy. I also suffered numerous respiratory infections as well as environmental allergies and chronic headaches. I frequently complained to my husband that my brain felt toxic. I never felt well.

My doctor prescribed Cipro (ciprofloxacin), yet another antibiotic. Days after I began taking it, my husband noticed a white patch on my cheek. I didn't give it much thought because I am so pale to begin with. A few months later, I began another round of Cipro. Within two days, I lost 30 percent of my pigmentation. White blotches covered my body. My dermatologist diagnosed me with vitiligo, an autoimmune disease that affects 1 to 2 percent of the population.

At this point, I had had enough of doctors who were bound to the Western tradition of medicine. I was determined to find a medical doctor who practiced alternative medicine.

The Turning Point

My first encounter with non-Western medical care was with the Traditional Chinese Medical (TCM) doctor, who succeeded in treating our ear infections by warning us to not consume dairy products.

At about that time, I had read *The Yeast Syndrome,* a book by John Parks Trowbridge and Morton Walker. It struck a chord. *Candida,* the book reported, could exhaust the endocrine system and lead to many conditions, including two I'd been diagnosed with: hypothyroidism and vitiligo. Frequent use of antibiotics could cause candidiasis, as could a diet like mine—one high in sugar.

It was difficult to find a physician who believed that candidiasis even existed, let alone one who knew how to treat it. I was finally referred to David Allen, a physician who practices both conventional and alternative medicine. In my first visit to his office, he explained that a pregnancy can deplete a woman's body of nutrients and send her immune system on a downward spiral. That made sense to me, especially as a mother of twins, whose behavior and health issues had put a lot of stress on my immune system.

I underwent several tests, including one for candidiasis, which indicated that my *Candida* levels were indeed high. Dr. Allen prescribed nystatin, an antifungal medicine. I went on an antifungal diet, which is no easy task, but I wanted to get well. To get rid of *Candida,* many foods must be eliminated from the diet, such as sugar, wheat, rye, dairy, mushrooms, alcohol, all junk food, refined food, artificial sweeteners, and fermented foods, like vinegar and soy sauce.

But my candidiasis wouldn't budge. If anything, it was getting worse. I took myself off nystatin after one year, but I didn't give up hope.

The Next Steps

Plagued with allergies, vitiligo, and Hashimoto's thyroid, I attended a medical lecture featuring a panel of doctors, one of whom spoke about autoimmune diseases and offered a warning that would change my life. "If you are in your thirties and forties and have been suffering from autoimmune diseases," he said, "it may be connected to the amalgam fillings in your mouth."

Amalgam fillings. One of my earliest memories involved going to the dentist—I had plenty of cavities. They were filled with amalgam, silvery metal containing mercury. By adulthood, I had fifteen mercury amalgam fillings in my mouth.

I never thought much about my metal filings until I was in my early twenties, when I began hearing a strange buzzing noise in my head as I fell asleep. It was scary, but I could stop the buzzing if I forced myself to wake up. As soon as I started to go back to sleep, the buzzing would return. I would try to wake back up, but I'd be too exhausted, almost as though I were paralyzed. I would awaken the next morning feeling okay but baffled by what had occurred.

One afternoon, as I lay down to nap, I again heard buzzing, but I decided not to fight the noise. To my surprise, I tuned into a radio station! The sound was clear and loud.

Befuddled, I told a friend about the experience. He speculated that the silver in my fillings was acting as an antenna, and I was picking up radio waves. I talked to my dentist, who confirmed that there were documented cases of amalgam fillings tuning into radio frequencies. The mystery was solved, and, coincidentally, the buzzing sound never returned.

After hearing the doctor's warning against amalgam fillings, it was clear that it was time to start thinking about my teeth again. The silver amalgams had been the culprit behind the mysterious buzzing in my head when I was in my twenties; could they also be behind the mystery of my impaired immune system? I had already read in alternative medicine books that mercury contributes to candidiasis. I knew I had to take action and figure out whether mercury was damaging my health.

Soon after the lecture, I had my body tested for heavy metals with the urine toxic element DMPS (dimethyl mercapto propionic acid) test. The results showed my mercury levels were in a highly elevated range. I never ate fish, so I knew my amalgam fillings were the source of the mercury poisoning in my body.

Over the next several months, I had all my fillings removed and replaced with composite material. I never again experienced another toxic headache. I later had several DMPS IVs (chelation therapy treatments) to help my body detoxify from the mercury.

Afterward, I began having fewer respiratory infections, and my environmental allergies no longer bothered me. My energy increased. I then began to take an antifungal medicine, Diflucan (fluconazole). Finally, after eight years of vitiligo, a significant amount of my skin's pigmentation returned.

About that time, Dr. Allen was testing Westley for amino acid deficiencies. A lack of amino acids in the diet, or difficulty digesting amino acids, could precipitate exactly the sort of attention and behavioral problems Westley had experienced for years. The test results showed that Westley's amino acid levels were indeed low. I wondered about Erik's levels, and my own. Sure enough, tests showed that our amino acid levels were low, too.

A compound pharmacy created a custom amino acid mix to address my exact deficiency. To help with metabolizing these amino acids, I took vitamin B$_6$. As with Erik and Westley, the results were amazing. Supplementing my diet with amino acids elevated my energy and general health to a level that I never before experienced. I found it much easier to focus and was able to better handle everyday stress. (For more information on supplements and laboratories that conduct tests for amino acids, heavy metals, pesticides, other toxins, and *Candida,* please see Resources, p. 179–181).

Why Me?

When I reflect on my childhood, I realize what likely caused my persistent illnesses and attention disorder. The amalgam fillings were one contributing factor. I also believe my poor diet, which once included far too much sugar, further hampered my health.

I was born with an insane addiction to sugar. My mother kept few sweets in the house; unfortunately, that did not stop me from making sugar the staple of my diet. I recall walking one mile to the corner store, when I was as young as seven years old, because a quarter would buy me five candy bars. I made sure that I ate them all before I got home so my mother would not find out about my sweet secret. Since then, I've learned a lot about sugar—particularly how it can encourage *Candida* growth and how it negatively affects mood, attention, and behavior.

Beyond the fillings and the sugar, I've concluded that the exposure to pesticides during my childhood also impaired my health. In the 1950s and 1960s, when I was growing up, trucks drove down our streets and sprayed insecticides on the trees to kill mosquitoes. I spent a lot of time as a young girl outside, climbing trees and exploring nature. I remember seeing pesticide residue dripping from the trees I climbed.

In exploring natural health issues, I have learned that some of the common symptoms of pesticide poisoning include an inability to think, poor concentration, hyperactivity, poor coordination, weakness, nervousness, breathing problems, muscle pains, and twitching—the symptoms we associate with a number of neurological challenges, including ADHD. Fortunately, in the 1960s, people became alarmed over the amount of insecticides being used and their effect on animals and people, thanks in large part to Rachel Carson's book *Silent Spring* (Houghton Mifflin Company, 1962). The U.S. government began to gradually phase out all uses of DDT in 1972. In 1975, most uses of chlordane were banned.

Staying Healthy

To get and stay well, I had to become proactive in educating myself. I read books on alternative medicine, attended lectures, and listened carefully to alternative medicine practitioners, all of which has led me to adopt the natural-living lifestyle.

To help detox from toxins, I use chlorella algae, which has been proven to bind with and remove toxic metals and pesticides from the body. I also use cilantro for detoxification purposes. To support my brain, adrenals, and thyroid, I take essential fatty acids such as flaxseed oil and evening primrose. I no longer take Synthroid because it is synthetic and often ineffective. Instead, I use a raw thyroid glandular supplement. To prevent recurring candidiasis, I take acidophilus to balance my intestinal flora and natural antifungal supplements, such as olive leaf extract.

I buy organic produce, and I eat raw food as much as possible. For breakfast, I mix two tablespoons of Dr. Schulze's Superfood in a glass of vegetable juice. Dr. Schulze's Superfood is 100 percent organic, made with whole food and herbal vitamins and minerals (see www.herbdoc.com). The ingredients are spirulina, blue-green algae, chlorella, alfalfa, barley, wheatgrass, purple dulse (a sea vegetable), beetroot, spinach, rosehips, orange peel, lemon peel, and inactive *Saccharomyces cerevisiae* nutritional yeast. Because Superfood is made of numerous single-celled microplants, the body is able to assimilate it in minutes, right into the bloodstream. I have not had one infection since supplementing my diet with Superfood.

The lesson I learned through my journey to get well is that there was no magic pill to cure me. I had to address many conditions to bring my body to a healthy state. Detoxifying from mercury and other toxins, along with major dietary changes, supplements (particularly amino acid supplements), and eating whole, vibrant food (rather than processed, lifeless food) made the difference.

Many seemingly irrelevant or unrelated factors, such as nutritional deficiencies, digestive disorders, candidiasis, artificial food coloring, artificial sweeteners, food allergies, heavy metal toxicity, environmental toxins, vaccines, mold, fungi, seizures, thyroid disorders, brain trauma, and electromagnetic field disturbances can cause symptoms of ADHD, autism, and other neurological problems.

To treat ADHD successfully, no stone should be left unturned; every possible root cause and natural solution should be accurately considered and assessed. By addressing the root causes of my children's and my symptoms through the removal of toxic foods from our diets, detoxification, and taking quality nutritional supplements, we succeeded on our journeys to healing.

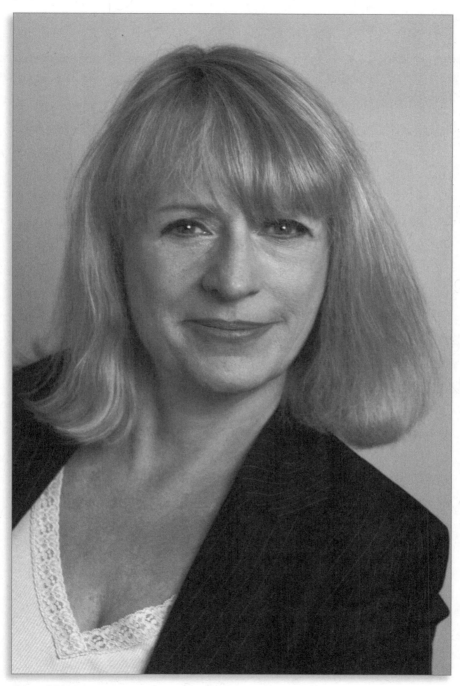

"You CAN have victory over ADHD—just like we did!"

Food Coloring, Toxic Metals, and Aspartame

Mark's Story

Looking back, it was a challenging road filled with highs and lows. There were many days I didn't have the time or energy to wear anything but sweatpants. Wearing makeup didn't even cross my mind; it was hard enough to get out of bed and face another day.

Fortunately, after countless hours of research and classes, hope and prayer, phenomenal practitioners who took a personal interest in Mark and our family, and most important the support of my husband, my older son Luke, my mother and sister, the transformation in Mark has been phenomenal. Close friends describe it as miraculous.

Here is my family's story and the path we took to help my son Mark recover from lead poisoning and some learning issues.

Our Lives for the Past Several Years

Misdiagnoses, labeling, specialist after specialist, frustration, guilt, blame, worry, crying, vomiting, infections, temper outbursts, a diet of chicken nuggets and pizza, therapy upon therapy, not enough hours in the day, marriage stress, financial pressure.

Our Lives Today

Correct diagnosis, public school, high IQ, play dates, soccer, basketball, piano, two dogs, green beans, peas, pancakes, some therapy, family vacations, happiness, smiles, laughter, peace.

The Symptoms

Mark was perpetually sick as a child. He had frequent infections, skin rashes, and bouts of vomiting, particularly after eating foods or taking medicines with red and yellow food coloring like Amoxicillin or Robitussin. He was diagnosed with asthma and would vacillate between being hyperactive and lethargic. He lost his clarity of speech and sometimes seemed to have a hard time understanding what we were saying. All of my friends with children commented that Mark seemed to be sick more than his fair share.

The Search for a Diagnosis

When Mark was eighteens months old, we pressed our pediatrician for answers, and he sent us for allergy testing. The allergist diagnosed Mark with asthma. At the time of the appointment, Mark happened to have yet another ear infection, so we started him on antibiotics. We treated his asthma with a nebulizer and medications provided by the allergist. The doctor thought that maybe Mark's coughing was causing him to vomit, so we followed through with the treatment. Mark still experienced the coughing, and we had to be sure not to get medications that were red or yellow, otherwise Mark would vomit. We eventually found a compounding pharmacy that could make the medications free of dye so Mark could ingest them without problems.

We were also concerned about Mark's speech, loss of some fine motor skills, and his lack of interest in food. We saw a neurologist several times and some psychologists. We received a variety of different diagnoses, some worse than others, but nothing really seemed to fit. All we knew was that our son was getting sicker and skinnier and just wasn't looking healthy.

The Turning Point

Years ago, my mother went through a similar situation. She was constantly fatigued, achy, had rashes and headaches, and just generally did not feel well. We went to so many physicians and eventually to a psychologist, who diagnosed her with anxiety and depression. We knew this was not this case but didn't have any answers. She just continued on with her struggle, and we tried to help her in every way possible.

Then, several years later, the company where I was working offered a wellness screening. I brought my mother in, and the test results revealed that her liver enzymes were extremely high. We phoned her physician, who referred us to a specialist. Finally, after years of searching for answers, Mom was diagnosed with hepatitis C.

Her story and perseverance kept us going through all of our challenges with Mark. She kept saying, "Don't give up. Do you remember when they told me it was in my head? Do you remember how sick I was and how you believed me?

Believe in what you see; believe in what Mark is showing you." We couldn't accept anything less than the truth.

Mark had yet another infection, and when we were at the pediatrician's office, I noticed a brochure about an ADHD drug, published by the manufacturer. Since ADHD was among the many labels that had been bandied about for Mark, I picked up the brochure and read it. The pharmaceutical company recommended screening for lead poisoning prior to starting the drug, because the symptoms of lead poisoning often resemble ADHD. I brought this up to the pediatrician, but she said it wasn't a concern in our case since we lived in a newer home.

We decided to keep searching for answers, and another friend referred us to another doctor. After examining Mark, the new doctor asked if we had ever considered whether lead poisoning or some other type of toxicity could be causing Mark's problems. We explained that we lived in a newer home and were told that was not a concern. He then ran a battery of tests. When we met with him at our next appointment, he told us that based on his screenings he was convinced Mark had lead poisoning. After testing our dinnerware and discovering it had lead, we purchased new plates and began a quest to determine what other contaminants were affecting Mark.

The Treatment

We started Mark on dimercaptosuccinic acid (DMSA), a drug approved by the Food and Drug Administration (FDA) for use in acute metal poisoning. (The trade name for DMSA is Chemet.) We started seeing improvements immediately. Mark's preschool teachers, therapists, and friends all commented on his progress. On the one hand we were deeply disturbed by the diagnosis; after all, the stories we had read about lead-poisoned children were fairly depressing. Nevertheless, we were determined to do anything to help our son.

The lead poisoning had greatly affected Mark's speech, plus he had developed auditory processing problems. Although his fine motor skills had previously been good, simple tasks, such as eating with a fork and drawing, had become challenging for him. So, in addition to the chelation therapy (DMSA), Mark was given occupational therapy, physical therapy, speech therapy, sauna therapy, homeopathy, acupuncture with BioSET (an allergy desensitization technique), and nutritional supplementation. By chance, we stumbled upon vibrational sound healing, and this therapy proved to be extremely beneficial for the entire family. Vibrational sound healing, along with wholesome, organic foods, provided the foundation for Mark's healing. We also participated in Interactive Metronome (IM) therapy (IM is a neuromotor assessment and treatment tool used to improve the neurological processes of motor planning and sequencing), HANDLE (a nondrug alternative for identifying and treating neurodevelopmental disorders; it draws on perspectives and techniques from a variety of disciplines), and began music lessons. Everyone played a part in Mark's healing.

The Results

When Mark was two and a half, a psychologist who assessed him informed us that he thought Mark's IQ was around 70. When I think of this now, it's a reminder of just how wrong some "experts" can be. The psychologist performed an IQ test on a sick child and then tried to determine his IQ. Incredibly, Mark's IQ went from 70 at that time to 128 today.

Mark had acquired many labels, but none were helpful or accurate. A lot of them were simply symptoms of his underlying illness—lead poisoning. Since lead poisoning can mimic or be misdiagnosed as ADHD, autism, auditory processing problems, or other learning disabilities, it is important to insist on a lead poisoning test from your physician. The sooner the lead is removed from the child's body, the better the prognosis.

At age seven, Mark is a happy, healthy boy who loves learning and school, takes piano lessons, plays a number of sports, eats well, and enjoys playing with friends and his dogs. He is truly full of joy. Mark still attends speech and occupational therapy, though not as often as he used to, and he continues to listen to vibrational sound healing CDs two to three times a week. We are so grateful to have found what works for him. We hope that by sharing his story and outlining potential therapies, we can help your child make great strides as well.

—Debbie Lindgren
President, bluedominoes, inc.
www.bluedominoes.com

> Because the symptoms of lead poisoning can mimic other childhood conditions, such as ADHD and autism, it is imperative that children be properly screened for lead poisoning prior to their diagnosis.
>
> - To learn more about the healing therapies mentioned in this article, visit www.bluedominoes.com/comp_healing.php.
>
> - For more information about wholesome, organic foods, visit www.bluedominoes.com/nutrition_recipes.php.
>
> - For more information regarding lead in plates, visit www.bluedominoes.com/ article_archive.php.

Artificial Food and Cosmetic Coloring

A HIDDEN SOURCE OF TOXIC METALS

Background

I rarely thought twice about food coloring—and when I did, I thought how wonderful it was. Isn't it great that you can make a green cake, decorate Easter eggs, customize treats for children, and make colorful play dough? It seemed as if every label I checked had some type of food coloring in it, so that meant it was safe, right? Unfortunately, the answer turned out to be a resounding No!

Why was it that some members of my family had a bad reaction after eating foods that contained coloring? Was it my imagination? Was it something else in the food? What about other children whose parents shared the same concern? Why did one child become hyperactive while another broke out in a rash? These questions haunted me, and I needed to find answers.

When we approached our pediatrician, she mentioned that some parents believe there is a connection between food coloring and behavior and illness; but she also said there was absolutely no evidence to support this. Because she couldn't provide any data to prove it wasn't detrimental, I decided to keep looking for answers. Eventually I heard of Ben Feingold, a pediatric allergist who made the link between diet, food coloring, and hyperactivity. A number of his patients improved or recovered by changing their diets, specifically by eliminating foods high in salicylates and those that contain colorings. Dr. Feingold had quite a bit of data on salicylates, but what really intrigued me was the link between food coloring and hyperactivity—what exactly was in these colors?

Artificial food colorings were first introduced after World War II, when the chemical industry joined with the food industry to introduce chemical-based colors, since they were lower in cost than natural colorings and had a longer shelf life. The safety of the artificial colors was determined primarily from using LD_{50} tests.

The LD_{50} is a standardized measure for expressing and comparing the toxicity of chemicals when tested on animals. The name refers to the dose that kills half (50 percent) of the animals tested (LD is an abbreviation for "lethal dose"). The animals typically used are rats, mice, rabbits, guinea pigs, and hamsters, among others, and the test results are then extrapolated to humans. At the time that artificial food colorings were approved, behavioral toxicology testing was not required by the FDA and therefore was not done.

The FDA and Food Colorings

The FDA's website is a valuable database for food coloring information. The site provides precise lists of color ingredients and is quite disturbing. I was horrified to learn that all artificial food colorings contain heavy metals, such as lead and mercury, as well as arsenic and myriad chemicals.

One reason this is so disturbing is that one area of the site contains information on the danger of lead contamination and its sources; however, food colorings are not listed as potential sources of exposure. This is especially frightening given all the possibilities for exposure to artificial food colorings in any given day. For example, does your child drink a sports drink or a fruit juice with coloring? Does his or her antibiotic contain coloring? What about the macaroni and cheese you made for dinner last night? What are the cumulative effects of this exposure?

Two colorings worth mentioning are not approved for food. The first color, Orange B, is authorized for use only in casings for hot dog and sausage casings. Were you aware that these foods had colorings in them? I certainly was not. Even if you are consciously trying to avoid colorings, you nevertheless have to be extremely vigilant and check every label, because colorings show up in very unexpected places like these.

The second color, Citrus Red No. 2, is approved only for orange skins that are not intended for or used in processing; this means the fresh oranges that we peel and eat. So although we may believe that oranges are a healthful fresh fruit, suitable to offer to our children, they are likely laced with heavy metals.

Cosmetic Colorings and Dermal Absorption

Artificial colorings are a major concern because not only are they in our food products, they are also present in other daily use items, such as lotions, shampoos, soaps, and cosmetics. Furthermore, the metal allotments for these products are even higher than those allowed in food products.

According to the Children's Environmental Health Project, dermal (skin) absorption is proportional to the concentration of the substance and the surface area to which the substance is applied. Dermal absorption rates vary from person to person and are affected by variables like skin thickness, occlusions, and the composition of the substance. If a substance is fat soluble, it will be more easily absorbed into the skin.

For these reasons, we must be as vigilant about what we put on our skin as we are about what we eat. In addition, because dermal absorption rates vary from person to person, and the amount of toxic substances vary from product to product, people will be affected differently by various products. Something as innocent as washing your hands with soap could expose you to more than you bargained for.

Several studies have been done on the dermal absorption of lead. One study concluded that significant amounts of inorganic lead compounds can be absorbed through the skin; therefore, protection should be used. Another study evaluated the effectiveness of skin cleansers at removing lead from the skin. The results show it's necessary to prevent skin contamination from occurring in the first place, because just brief contact allows for penetration, even when it is quickly followed by washing.

A page from history refutes the prevalent belief that topical products are not absorbed into the body through the skin. Mercurial ointments were used as a treatment for syphilis before the discovery of penicillin. The ointments were applied directly to the thinnest areas of the skin, such as the groin and the bends of the elbows and knees. Some scientists believed that the dermal absorption of the ointment was quite low and that patients were actually receiving benefit from inhaling the mercury vapor. A study was performed where the ointment was rubbed in and any excess was washed off the skin, eliminating any source of mercury vapor. Seventy-five percent of the study participants experienced salivation—one of the known effects of mercury—proving that dermal absorption played a key role.

According to the Department of Health and Human Services, dermal absorption of arsenic is low; however, it is readily absorbed if inhaled or ingested. Many wood-based playground structures were removed out of fears that children would touch the arsenic-treated wood and then put their hands in their mouths.

Colorings and Mental Health

As mentioned previously, Dr. Feingold identified a link between food colorings and hyperactivity. He also noticed a marked increase in ADD/ADHD classifications after the mass introduction of food colorings into our society. A brochure by McNeil Consumer & Specialty Pharmaceuticals, available in my pediatrician's office, indicates that lead exposure can lead to ADHD, yet the authors of the brochure discredit the idea that food and cosmetic colorings play any role in affecting children's behavior. If lead has been implicated in ADHD, and colorings have lead in them, then removing added colorings from our diets and environment is crucial.

The *Journal of Developmental & Behavioral Pediatrics* published information regarding fifteen trials with 219 participants; all were double-blind, crossover trials. Just by eliminating artificial food colorings from their diets, children's behavior improved significantly. Furthermore, just eliminating food colorings from the diet produced one-third to one-half the improvement typically seen with ADHD medication therapy. Even if one elects to use medication, heavy metal toxicity screenings need to be prescribed prior to taking psychoactive drugs, because most of these drugs contain colorings that can lead to further toxicity.

Colorings in ADHD Medications

I t is instructive to consider how saturated with artificial colorings most ADHD medications are. For example, Ritalin contains D&C Yellow No. 10; Strattera contains FD&C Blue No. 2, synthetic iron oxide, and edible black ink; and Dexedrine contains FD&C Yellow No. 5 and No. 6.

Children taking these drugs are being exposed to lead, arsenic, and mercury, among many other toxins. Parents also need to be extremely careful with whatever medications they may give their children, including acetaminophen, ibuprofen, and antibiotics, and ensure that alternative products don't contain food dyes. As parents, we can check food labels, but we must rely on our physicians to select our medicines, since the bottles provided by the pharmacist don't list all of the ingredients. Colloidal silver, homeopathic products, and supplements may provide a safer alternative.

Several studies also point to a link between lead poisoning and ADHD. One of the most recent was published in the journal *Environmental Health Perspectives*. The study results showed that children with blood lead levels of more than 2 micrograms of lead per deciliter were four times more likely to be diagnosed with ADHD than children with levels below 0.8 micrograms per deciliter. The acceptable blood level for lead, according to the government, is 10 micrograms per deciliter. The study estimates that more than five million children between the ages of four and fifteen in the United States have levels higher than 2 micrograms per deciliter.

Another study performed by the National Academy of Sciences (NAS) in 2000 contends that roughly 3 percent of all developmental and neurological disorders in the United States are caused by toxic chemicals and other environmental contaminants. The same study showed that environmental triggers, along with a genetic predisposition, may cause approximately 25 percent of developmental and neurological deficits. The NAS also acknowledged that the study was only referring to well-recognized and clinically diagnosed mental and physical disabilities, and therefore the 25 percent estimate may in fact be higher.

What Is Your Child Exposed to on a Daily Basis?

M ost parents I speak to are completely unaware of the coloring content of their food, cosmetic products, and medicines. Some who are aware are shocked to find out that colorings do not come from natural substances.

Here are some surprising examples of food and personal care products you might use that contain food colorings:

- Bathtime Colorblast Tablets: FD&C Blue No. 1, D&C Red No. 33, FD&C Yellow No. 5

- Flintstones Vitamins: aspartame, FD&C Red No. 40 Al Lake, FD&C Yellow 6 Al Lake, FD&C Blue No. 2

- Gatorade Fruit Punch: Red No. 40

- Johnson's Baby Shampoo: D&C Yellow No. 10 and D&C Orange No. 4

- M&Ms (plain): Blue No. 1, Blue No. 1 Lake, Blue No. 2 Lake, Red No. 40, Red No. 40 Lake, Yellow No. 5, Yellow No. 6

- Pampers Hand Soap: Yellow No. 5, Green No. 5, Orange No. 4

- Tylenol Plus Cold Infant Drops: Red No. 33, Red No. 40

We do not know the cumulative effects of regular exposure to food and cosmetic colorings and lead, mercury, and arsenic. We also do not know how food colorings interact with each other and with other toxic substances. I have found no studies regarding this, and that alone is alarming.

Cleaning products present an interesting challenge, since manufacturers do not have to identify the ingredients of their products on the labels. Material Safety Data Sheets (MSDS) are available for consumers to view via most companies' websites. Although manufacturers are required to provide information on the MSDS regarding established exposure limits, they are not required to provide an ingredient list because their formulations are protected by patent laws.

The Effects of Lead, Mercury, and Arsenic

Lead

We've all heard that lead poisoning is associated with lower IQ, but did you know it could also be responsible for some cavities? According to a study published in the *Journal of the American Medical Association* (June 23/30; 281:2294), where data from 24,901 children was analyzed, a correlation between lead and cavities was established. Most of the children participating in the study had blood lead levels of only a few micrograms of lead per deciliter—well below the federal guideline for blood-lead concentrations of 10 mcg per deciliter. For children age five to seventeen, an increased burden of 5 mcg per deciliter of blood corresponded to an 80 percent increase in cavities. The researchers estimate that cavities of 2.7 million U.S. children result from lead poisoning, about 10 percent of all cases in that age group. The researchers speculate that either lead stunts development of the glands that produce saliva (which protects teeth from harmful acid and bacteria) or lead might hinder enamel growth.

The American Academy of Child and Adolescent Psychiatry estimates that one out of every six children in the United States has blood lead levels in the toxic range. Lead exposure has been linked to developmental delays, peripheral neuropathy, altered thyroid hormone, and reduced fertility. In elderly adults, levels over 4 mcg can have neurobehavioral effects.

Mercury

So what happens when we get a cavity? Some dentists will fill our teeth with amalgams that contain mercury. Mercury has been implicated in autism, ADHD, learning disabilities, endocrine problems, allergies, asthma, rheumatoid arthritis, and a host of other disorders. According to the FDA, "The toxicity of mercury compounds is extensively documented in scientific literature. It is well known that mercury compounds are readily absorbed through unbroken skin as well as through the lungs by inhalation and by intestinal absorption after ingestion. Mercury is absorbed from topical application and is accumulated in the body, giving rise to numerous adverse effects... Recently it has also been determined that microorganisms in the environment can convert various forms of mercury into highly toxic methyl mercury, which has been found in the food supply and is now considered to be a serious environmental problem."

Common Dreams newswire reported in 2004 that Environmental Protection Agency scientists using data collected by the Centers for Disease Control estimated that one in six pregnant women has enough mercury in her blood to pose a risk of brain damage to her developing child. Lower levels of mercury can lead to a variety of symptoms, including fever, insomnia, rapidly changing moods, and tremors.

Arsenic

Arsenic poisoning has been linked to respiratory, neurological, developmental, and cardiovascular issues. It has also been associated with cancer. In fact, an increased risk of skin cancer in humans has been connected with chronic exposure to inorganic arsenic in medication, contaminated water, and the workplace.

Arsenic is present in foods such as meat, fish, and poultry and, according to the Department of Health and Human Services, our dietary intake accounts for 80 percent of our exposure (although fish arsenic has a low toxicity in humans and is excreted rapidly in our urine). Fungicides, herbicides, insecticides, paints, and water are other sources of arsenic exposure.

A study of 201 children under the age of ten concluded that as little as .0017 mg of arsenic per day affected children's performance in tasks that required switching attention. When the exposure increased to .0034 mg per day, the children showed decreased performance in tasks that involved switching attention as well as in tests that measured memory.

What Can We Do?

The first step is to remove colorings from our environment. Although this might appear difficult because colorings are so pervasive, there are easy options and alternatives. For example, if you want to color a cake frosting or home-made play dough, look in your natural food store for packaged colorings made from real food such as turmeric, blueberries, or beets. You can also make your own natural colorings by adding these foods to whatever it is you want to dye. Natural food stores also carry a variety of foods, personal care products, non-prescription medications, and cleaners that do not contain colorings.

Preparing as many meals as possible from scratch at home is also a step in the right direction, because that way you can control what you put in your food. If you need to obtain medication and are not sure if it contains colorings, you can check online at www.rxlist.com. If your medication is made with colorings, contact a compounding pharmacy to see if the pharmacist can compound it without the added colors. A list of compounding pharmacies can be found at www.iacprx.org.

—Debbie Lindgren
President, bluedominoes, inc.
www.bluedominoes.com

ADHD by Any Other Name

Not only is the handwriting on the wall, it's scrawled all over our children: Chemicals are hurting us! Hyperactivity has existed since humankind began, but it hasn't always been called the same thing. Various names have been used in the past to describe attention deficit hyperactivity disorder (ADHD) and they are not all bad—think of labels such as enthusiastic, creative, nonconformist, daydreamer, eccentric, high-energy, dedicated, obsessive, type A personality.

So why the name change? No particular reason really. The American Psychiatric Association publishes the official guidelines for naming and diagnosing mental disorders. Their reference book *Diagnostic and Statistical Manual of Mental Disorders* is regularly updated as scientists deal more and more with unidentified modern diseases. Research in the late 1980s began to show changes in "attention deficit," so it was simply renamed for more modern times.

To date, no one has identified the cause for this "mental alteration." Here is yet another example of an increasing health symptom (particularly among children) with no known cause or cure. Once again, it's time to examine our modern diet of chemical sweeteners and food additives for the mental influences they have on human behavior.

Can ADHD be caused by artificial sweeteners? You bet. Just look around. The increases in ADHD (and the label itself) are perfectly timed with the introduction of the artificial sweetener aspartame (in such products as NutraSweet and Equal) in 1981. After over twenty years of use, and now with the current blending of artificial sweeteners, I predict the impact of this already existing problem will continue climbing to devastating levels.

There is no simple test, like a blood test or a written test, to determine whether a child has ADHD. This is true of many medical conditions; for example, there is no "test" for a simple headache, yet anyone who has had a headache knows it's real. Usually in these cases, the health symptoms are a reaction to a cause that cannot be seen—a chemical cause, such as artificial sweeteners.

I have many clients with obvious health symptoms—headaches, sleeplessness, numbness in their arms and legs, vertigo, depression—but no medical tests previously done, such as MRIs, CAT scans, or blood or urine tests, show any physical reason for their symptoms. Most traditional medical doctors are puzzled by this but simply blame the symptoms on stress, prescribe medication, and send the patient home to deal with it. If only they knew to look at their patients' diets and the amount of artificial sweeteners they use as a probable cause. The same scenario occurs when children are diagnosed with and treated for ADHD, when they are merely reacting to artificial sweeteners or other food additives. In both situations, the patient is left with no answers and a lot of frustration.

According to a June 1997 American Medical Association study, "ADHD is one of the best researched disorders in medicine, and the overall data on its validity are far more compelling than that for most mental disorders and even for many medical conditions." One of the best researched disorders they state, yet the cause remains elusive to traditional medicine. What's wrong with this picture? It's time to recognize artificial chemical sweeteners as one of the root causes of ADHD, and we need to offer these kids the proper help they need. No more drugs, no more ostracizing, and above all, no more artificial sweeteners!

In this ever-continuing web of confusion over which chemicals are causing which health reactions, it is best to return to natural sweeteners and whole foods, especially during pregnancy and during childhood development. It is always better to be safe than sorry when it comes to our children.

Diana Dow-Edwards of SUNY Health Science Center in Brooklyn investigated evidence of mental retardation and developmental disabilities in laboratory guinea pigs by administering aspartame to them during pregnancy. Since brain development occurs in the womb in both guinea pigs and humans, the results of her investigations could be extrapolated to people.

Dow-Edwards' research evaluated the harmful influences of moderate doses of aspartame administered to pregnant mothers, especially those with liver problems, because all chemical sweeteners are metabolized in the liver. She concluded from her studies that using moderate quantities of aspartame during pregnancy could produce a dramatic increase in the number of offspring born with diminished brain function. Not only does this study call into question the use of aspartame, but it also challenges the use of sweetener blends, such as those that combine aspartame and sucralose. Where aspartame penetrates, so follows the chlorine in sucralose. Corporate marketers claim that the chlorine atoms in sucralose (which goes by the brand name Splenda) are so tightly bound they do not break down inside the body, but when sucralose is blended with aspartame, the chlorine in sucralose can be ushered into the brain alongside its chemical counterpart.

As early as 1970, John Olney, a research psychiatrist in the Department of Psychiatry at Washington School of Medicine, pioneered proof of aspartame's dangerous entry into the brain. He informed G. D. Searle Pharmaceuticals (the developer of aspartame and founder of The NutraSweet Company), warning them that the aspartic acid in aspartame caused holes to form in the brains of his laboratory mice. Olney proved that excess aspartic acid in the brain destroys brain neurons. He established that approximately 75 percent of the neural cells in any particular area of the brain could be killed before any clinical symptoms of a chronic illness are even noticed. "Neural cell damage can occur from excessive aspartic acid allowing too much calcium into the cells, triggering excessive amounts of free radicals, which kill brain cells," Olney stated.

Russell L. Blaylock, a professor of neurosurgery at the Medical University of Mississippi, provides over 500 scientific references in his book *Excitotoxins: The Taste That Kills*, proving that excess free excitatory amino acids (such as the aspartic acid and phenylalanine found in aspartame) cause serious chronic neurological disorders along with a host of acute physical symptoms. "The risk to infants, children, pregnant women, the elderly, and people with certain chronic health problems caused by excitotoxins is great," he writes.

The Federation of American Societies for Experimental Biology states, "The existence of evidence of potential responses to aspartame between males and females suggests a neuroendocrine link, and should be avoided by women of childbearing age and by individuals with affective disorders."

The FDA has recorded in their files the following mental symptoms related to aspartame use: depression, anxiety attacks, fatigue and malaise, sleep problems, vision problems, headaches and migraines. The evidence is clear that artificial sweeteners negatively affect the human brain. Before you commit your child to toxic medications to control bad behavior, try eliminating the toxic chemicals in their diet first. You might be pleasantly surprised at the results.

—Janet Starr Hull, PhD

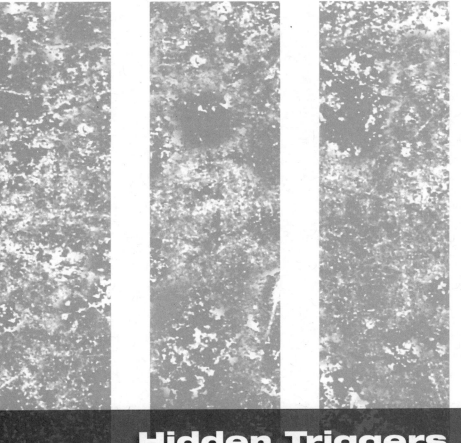

Hidden Triggers

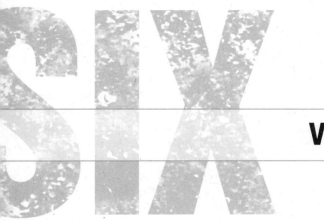

CHAPTER 6

Vaccinations

A PARENT'S RIGHT TO CHOOSE

T he vaccine decision is one of the most important choices we make as parents. Increasingly, childhood vaccines are implicated as the cause of growing rates of autism and ADHD. However, in questioning vaccines, we open ourselves up to a great deal of criticism, disapproval, and accusations of child neglect from doctors, school administrators, public health officials, family members, and other parents. How, they ask, do we dare question a practice that has prevented so many devastating diseases and saved so many lives? Aren't we putting our child and other children at risk for contracting serious diseases? After all, the government agencies designated to protect public health and most doctors say that childhood vaccines are safe.

If you dig a little deeper into the issue, you'll find many gaps and limitations in the data and knowledge regarding vaccine safety. Vaccines *are* capable of causing serious damage. Because they contain lab-altered viruses, bacteria, and toxic substances, vaccines have the ability to cause mild to severe neurological and immune damage or even death, depending on the vaccine given, the combination of vaccines given, the health of the child at the time of vaccination, and the genetic or biological factors that predispose the child to this damage. Vaccines are potent and toxic drugs that contain formaldehyde, mercury, aluminum, antibiotics, and other toxic components. Thoughtful parents are beginning to question the practice of injecting these toxic substances into the bodies of small babies and artificially manipulating their fragile immune systems during the crucial time of brain and immune development.

No Long-Term or Real-World Safety Studies

P harmaceutical companies do safety testing of vaccines, but long-term studies are not done. The follow-up for vaccine safety testing on individuals before a vaccine is marketed is only a few weeks or a couple of months at the most. Pharmaceutical companies and government health officials rely on post-marketing data to see if there are reports of serious side effects and reactions after the vaccine has been released and given to millions of children. But most doctors are reluctant to report adverse reactions, and it is estimated that only between 1 and 10 percent of vaccine reactions are ever reported. Even so, between 12,000 and 14,000 adverse reactions (including hospitalizations, injuries, and death) are reported annually to the Vaccine Adverse Event Reporting System (VAERS). Since it may be difficult to establish causal relationship, many of the reported reactions are dismissed as coincidental with no further study.

The control groups for determining adverse reactions are not unvaccinated children. Instead, they are children who have received other vaccines. This makes it possible for the vaccine in question to appear safer than it actually may be. In addition, no adequate studies have ever been done on the real-world risk—the cumulative effect of multiple doses of numerous vaccines given in the first five years of life.

Chronic Diseases Rise as Vaccinations Increase

C hronic diseases and disabilities in children have risen dramatically as vaccination rates for a growing number of vaccines climb higher than ever before. Twenty-five years ago, children following the recommended vaccine schedule received twenty-three doses of seven vaccines before age six. Today's children get forty-eight doses of fourteen vaccines by age six. With the additional recommendation for annual flu shots, children may now get sixty-nine doses of sixteen vaccines by age eighteen.

Given all these vaccinations, are our children healthier? In 1983, one in ten thousand American children was diagnosed with autism. Currently, one in every one hundred fifty children is diagnosed with autism. One out of six American children is considered learning disabled. One in nine has asthma, and one in four hundred fifty is diabetic. In 2003, almost four and a half million children were reported to have attention deficit and hyperactivity, and this chronic condition is on the increase.

Health officials continue to insist that there is no connection between vaccines and autism. However, Bernadine Healy, former head of the National Institutes of Health and a member of the Institute of Medicine, has stated that public health officials have intentionally avoided researching the link between vaccines and autism because they are afraid the answer will scare the public. She acknowledges that public health officials have failed to fully research vaccines and how they may contribute to autism. Dr. Healy, along with many other medical doctors, believes there may be a subset of children who, for genetic or other reasons, are susceptible to developing autism following vaccination.

In fact, the U.S. government has recently conceded in "vaccine court" that vaccines contributed to the development of autism in a child who is now age nine. There are thousands more autism cases in line to be heard in court in which the parents believe that vaccines contributed to their children's autism.

In June 2007, the first-ever investigation to determine the difference between vaccinated and unvaccinated children was done by Generation Rescue, a parent-funded nonprofit organization. This survey of over seventeen thousand children compared the rates of ADHD, autism, and asthma between vaccinated and unvaccinated children. Results showed that vaccinated U.S. children have a significantly higher risk of neurological disorders—including autism and ADHD—than unvaccinated children. This was not a comprehensive enough study to confirm a connection, but it certainly raises a big red flag and demonstrates the need for a national study to compare outcomes between vaccinated and unvaccinated children.

Toxicity of Vaccines

A growing number of doctors believe that a baby's immune system is not strong enough to handle the amount of vaccines typically given, and their livers and kidneys are not developed enough to metabolize or excrete the toxic chemicals and heavy metals in vaccines. Parents should know that even though mercury has finally been taken out of most childhood vaccines, there is still a significant amount of mercury in many flu shots as well as tetanus booster shots and some meningitis vaccines. Trace amounts of mercury still remain in other vaccines. Mercury is known to be one of the most toxic substances on Earth, and no amount of mercury is safe, especially when injected into a baby's small, developing body.

Even though most of the recent discussion concerning toxicity of vaccines has revolved around the mercury issue, mercury is certainly not the only toxicity problem with childhood vaccines. Aluminum is used as an adjuvant to boost the immune response of vaccines. Scientific evidence of the safety of injected aluminum is sorely lacking. Aluminum is a heavy metal that can accumulate in tissues and build up to toxic levels in the bloodstream, bones, and brain. Accumulation of aluminum in the brain is known to impair neurological and mental development. Animal studies show that aluminum causes convulsions, impaired memory, and defective learning.

The difference in the amount of aluminum that may be considered safe for babies and the amount that is actually contained in vaccines is alarming. The FDA website says that premature babies receiving injected aluminum through intravenous fluids at levels greater than 4 to 5 micrograms per kilogram of body weight per day can accumulate aluminum at levels associated with central nervous system and bone toxicity, and toxic buildup may occur at even lower rates. For a tiny premature baby, the toxic dose would be 10 to 20 mcg. It is estimated that a twelve-pound, two-month-old, full-term healthy baby could safely receive at least 30 mcg of intravenously injected aluminum per day. But it is unknown how much more aluminum a healthy baby could handle and how much could be safely injected into a baby via vaccines. The safety of aluminum in vaccines has never been established. No research has been done to determine a baby's ability to excrete aluminum to prevent toxic buildup. No one has measured the levels of aluminum absorption by the bloodstream when an aluminum-containing vaccine is injected into a baby. Also disturbing is the lack of data to determine if injected aluminum interacts with other vaccine toxins to cause harm to small, developing bodies.

A newborn baby receiving a hepatitis B shot on his first day of life gets 250 mcg of aluminum from this vaccine. The total amount of aluminum that a two-month-old baby receives from the recommended "well-baby" vaccines could vary from 295 mcg to 1,225 mcg, depending on which vaccines are given. This dose is usually repeated at four months and again at six months of age.

Vaccines also contain various animal products and are created using both human and animal tissues. These tissues can contain viruses and other contaminants. Even though there are processes to detoxify and clean the vaccines, some viruses have still made it into the final vaccine products that were injected into babies. One well-known case was a monkey virus known to cause cancer that was found in the polio vaccine given to millions of babies during the '50s and '60s. There remains a possibility of an unknown or new virus that may not be detected with current testing.

Vaccine Reactions

Vaccine reactions can take many forms, including one or more of the following:

- brain inflammation
- bruising
- collapse and/or shock
- death
- difficulty breathing or wheezing
- dizziness
- excessive sleepiness or lack of responsiveness
- high fever
- hives
- itching
- mental and/or physical regression
- muscle weakness or limpness
- paleness or changes in skin or lip color
- prolonged crying (especially high-pitched screaming in infants)
- rapid heart beat
- rash
- seizures or convulsions (shaking, twitching, jerking)
- swelling, redness, and pain at the injection site
- unusual irritability or other behavior changes
- vomiting or diarrhea

Many parents have reported that their baby had a high-pitched scream for many hours directly after receiving a vaccine and then regressed developmentally, eventually being diagnosed with autism months later. Some babies have died after being vaccinated.

Weakened Immunity

A growing number of doctors agree that weakened immunity and susceptibility to allergies, asthma, and chronic infections is another long-term consequence of the large number of vaccines given to babies and children at their most vulnerable time of immune development. A baby's immune system develops through breastfeeding and proper nutrition, and from its complex responses to natural exposure to disease. When a baby is naturally exposed to a virus, the immune system has several layers of responses that deal with the invasion. Allowing the range of acute inflammatory responses to typical childhood diseases strengthens immunity and strengthens the child's health overall.

Conversely, injecting multiple doses of altered viruses and toxins directly into the body bypasses many of the normal immune responses. The vaccine injection triggers antibody production, but antibodies are only one level of protection and not full natural immunity. The immune system is very complex, and the different branches of the immune system require a balanced, synergistic relationship to function properly. Repeated vaccinations may overstimulate the branch that produces antibodies, while suppressing the branch responsible for acute inflammatory responses.

Intelligent doctors and parents are beginning to question this manipulation of the immune system. Since we are seeing a huge increase in pediatric allergies, asthma, autoimmune diseases, and chronic immune deficiencies, we must look at a mass vaccination policy and demand the proper studies to find out what is happening to our children's immune systems.

Universal Vaccines for Everyone?

D oes it make sense to mandate vaccines for every child given the risks involved? The public health strategy for eliminating diseases includes universal vaccines for everyone, regardless of risks to the individual child, who may have biological or genetic susceptibility to vaccine damage. There are no tests that can show which babies will have serious reactions. Some children must be sacrificed in order to achieve the goal of eradicating disease in a population. They tell us that more lives will be lost to the disease if we don't vaccinate against it. But is this statement really true in the current reality of high-tech medicine in a population with effective sanitation and knowledge about the immunology of breastfeeding?

We cannot wipe out every disease on the planet. It may be more sensible to focus on naturally strengthening our children's immune systems to effectively deal with the increasing number of superbugs created by the inappropriate and massive use of antibiotics than to inject numerous toxins into their delicate, developing bodies. If we allow our children's immunity to develop on its own as nature intended, breastfeed, and use good nutrition and other natural immune-enhancing methods to keep our children's immunity strong, then why would we want to inject foreign material and toxins into their bodies that can weaken their health, especially since safety has not been proven? An increasing number of parents are not willing to take the risk of sacrificing their children to a point of view that goes against their core beliefs about health and wellness.

The Captive, Multibillion-Dollar Vaccine Market

What fuels the ubiquitous belief that vaccines are the supreme solution to disease and that those who do not accept vaccines are putting themselves and others at risk? In America's money-driven vaccine campaign, the vaccine industry uses the government, doctors, and school officials to effectively market their products and gain mass acceptance of their message. The Food and Drug Administration (FDA) accepts safety data from the manufacturers and licenses vaccines used in the United States. After a vaccine is licensed, the Advisory Committee on Immunization Practices (ACIP), appointed by the Centers for Disease Control (CDC), makes recommendations on dosages and age range for children. ACIP immunization recommendations are extremely influential and enacted into law as mandates by individual states. In the past twenty-five years, every childhood vaccine produced by the drug companies has been mandated for use by all American children.

Many members of both the ACIP and the FDA's advisory committees have been found by the U.S. Government Reform Committee to have blatant conflicts of interest, with strong financial ties to the pharmaceutical companies that make vaccines. The Government Reform Committee exposed these conflicts of interest, focusing on the approval of the rotavirus vaccine, which was found to cause severe bowel obstructions.

This vaccine was pulled from the market after a significant number of babies were injured and required surgery, and one baby died from the vaccine. It was found that the FDA's advisory committee members who approved the rotavirus vaccine were aware of the problems but voted to approve it anyway. Three out of these five members had financial ties to the pharmaceutical companies that were developing different versions of the rotavirus vaccine. This is not an isolated incident. Congressman Burton, the head of the Reform Committee, remarked, "If the panels that have made the decisions on all vaccines on the Childhood Immunization Schedule had as many conflicts as we found with rotavirus, then the entire process has been polluted and the public trust has been violated."

A mandate for every child in the country to use their vaccines gives the manufacturers a steady and constant demand for their products. And since they are protected from legal action by the Vaccine Injury Compensation Program of 1986, they are rushing to bring new vaccines to market. Vaccines are the only commercial products marketed and sold for profit in the United States that are not subject to product liability laws. It is predicted that the pediatric vaccine market will be more than $16 billion by the year 2016.

As more parents are beginning to mistrust vaccines, money is being spent to fund pro-vaccine organizations for public relations and damage control. Vaccine "experts" are hired to manipulate public opinion by denying the severity of adverse reactions and reinforcing the belief that the benefits of vaccines outweigh the risks. Instead of becoming alarmed by reports of vaccine-induced brain damage and pushing for the unbiased research needed to determine why this is happening, vaccine manufacturers and government agencies embark on intensive public relations campaigns to make sure the public trust in vaccines has not been diminished in any way. Their main goal is to keep the vaccine program moving forward at any cost. As author Randall Neustaedter warns parents in his *The Vaccine Guide: Making an Informed Choice*, "Vaccines represent consumer goods—and parents should research this product far more carefully than other purchases because their children's lives could be at stake."

Parents Can Make Informed Choices

A t the doctor's office, parents are given a two-page "Vaccine Information Statement," which highlights the importance of vaccines and downplays the harmful effects. Many parents are coerced into vaccinating their children by doctors who say they will no longer accept their children as patients if they are not vaccinated. Many parents are also worried that their children will be denied school attendance if they don't vaccinate.

Informed consent means that an informed patient (or parent) has absolute freedom to accept or reject any specific medical treatment or procedure. The patient (or parent) has the right to be treated sensitively and compassionately while learning about his or her options. The doctor is both ethically obligated and legally required to participate in a communication process that helps the patient to understand the risks and benefits as well as become aware of alternatives. There are informed consent statutes and case laws in all fifty states in the United States. Why don't these revered informed consent laws apply when it comes to vaccinations, especially when this medical intervention carries the risk of brain damage and death? Parents are almost never told about exemptions to state vaccine laws. They are usually told they do not have a choice.

The Association of American Physicians and Surgeons is deeply concerned that vaccine policy is based on incomplete studies of efficacy. They are also worried about the potential adverse effects of the vaccines and the violation of informed consent. "While we acknowledge that vaccines in the past have prevented many serious illnesses, they also have the potential to do great harm if given to the wrong individual," says the association's executive director Jane Orient. "That decision must be made by the patient in consultation with their physician—not through coercion by a government agency or school district."

We have the right to select the kind of preventive health care that is appropriate for our families. We should never be forced to accept any medical procedure that carries the risk of injury or death against our will. Making an informed decision requires that we evaluate the needs of our families and assess the pros and cons of each vaccine within this context. If we wish to take the precautionary approach and keep our children's bodies free from harmful toxins to develop healthy immunity naturally, we have every right to say no to vaccines.

In the United States, we have the legal right to exempt our children from vaccines in order for them to attend public school. All states have medical exemptions (these must be signed by a doctor), forty-eight states have exemptions for religious beliefs, and fifteen states have exemptions for philosophical beliefs. Claiming the philosophical exemption in some states (California, for example) is as easy as signing the statement on the back of the school's vaccination record or providing a letter that states that vaccinations are against your personal beliefs. When you claim an exemption, there should be no questions and your child legally must be admitted to school. A religious exemption can be a little trickier, sometimes requiring a letter from a recognized church, but in many cases parents can write a letter simply stating that vaccinations are against their religious beliefs.

If you are seeking an exemption, get a copy of your state's immunization law and follow exactly what it says about what is needed for an exemption. Many parents are not aware that these exemptions exist, since public health officials, doctors, and school administrators usually don't mention them.

We need to realize that our parental rights have been taken away in the process of trying to eradicate disease, in a way that can have devastating consequences to our children's health and well-being. We blindly put our faith in the medical industry and public health officials, who view disease as an enemy to exterminate at all costs, regardless of the number of damaged children or deaths that may occur in the process. When we accept these policies, we give our power over to the government and vaccine industry, and let them intrude in our family's private health care choices.

We, as parents, need to take our power back and make informed choices for our children without coercion, threat, or disapproval by doctors or health officials. And we should be applauded, not shamed, by our friends, family, and other parents for refusing to blindly follow "doctors' orders" as we carefully consider all the issues that can affect the health of our precious children. In fact, thorough investigation before making vaccine decisions and parental demand for proven safety is the *only* thing that will ever begin to make disease prevention safe for everyone's children.

—Jane Sheppard

Autism

THE MISDIAGNOSIS OF
OUR FUTURE GENERATIONS

O ver the last fifteen years, the incidence of autism has rapidly increased more than 5,700 percent in industrialized nations, from approximately 1 child in 10,000 in 1990 to 1 child out of 166. The United States and the United Kingdom have seen the sharpest rise. In some states, the incidence is now 1 child in 80, and we now have over 1.5 million children diagnosed with autism in the United States.

There's been a lot of attention regarding the link between mercury and autism, with mercury being the possible underlying factor. The issue of whether mercury plays a role in autism or other problems of the nervous system has been the subject of long debate among medical professionals, but now the evidence is overwhelmingly obvious.

This leads to the inevitable question: How do we get exposed to mercury? The sources surround us: mercury amalgams in our teeth, contamination of our water sources, the fish we consume, pollution from fossil fuels, breast milk, and virtually all vaccinations, just to name a few. If mercury is so devastating, why is it allowed to be in our flu shots, other vaccines, foods, and more? This is the million-dollar question, although it is quite evident to the well informed that the answer will be found somewhere along the money trail. Mercury is an inexpensive ingredient and has been used for so long that its removal now would be an admission of guilt on the part of vaccine manufacturers.

Mercury Exposure from
Vaccines and Other Sources

Many vaccines contain a substance called thimerosal, a preservative that contains mercury. Increased exposure to mercury from the thimerosal in vaccines is one of the most important issues relative to the increase in autism. Thimerosal is converted to ethyl mercury (a substance that is reportedly hundreds of times, and possibly a thousand times, more destructive than inorganic mercury) in less than one minute after being introduced into the body. This should give great concern to those appointed to protect the public, yet it is virtually ignored. Why is this highly toxic substance still allowed to be an ingredient of vaccines used to inoculate our precious children, our own future generations?

As far back as July 13, 1991, the vaccine manufacturer Eli Lilly documented on their own letterhead that thimerosal is "a product containing a chemical known to the State of California to cause birth defects or other reproductive harm." The company states in this document that mercury exposure can cause skin allergies, vision problems, and numbness in adults and mild to severe mental retardation and mild to severe impairment to motor coordination in children. Yet Eli Lilly continues to use thimerosal in the manufacturing of vaccines. Furthermore, we inoculate our children starting the day they are born, introducing multiple vaccines with higher and higher amounts of mercury (thimerosal) into their vulnerable and delicate bodies.

However, the vaccine issue must not overshadow problems caused by the cumulative exposure to mercury from all sources experienced by children before birth and during early infancy. These additional exposures include but are certainly not limited to mercury in foods, amalgam fillings in teeth (which contribute greatly to the amount of mercury in a pregnant mother's system), RhoGAM (immunoglobulin) given to mothers during pregnancy, tetanus shots, pollution from fossil fuels, water contamination, and mercury compounds used in skin products.

There is absolutely no reason for the use of a mercury-based preservative in human vaccines. Even the American Veterinary Society had thimerosal removed from animal vaccinations over fifteen years ago because of the known toxicity of mercuric compounds. Unfortunately, as a society we are virtually ignorant to the severe biological burden that mercury places on our bodies.

Each year the government conducts the National Health and Nutrition Examination Survey (NHANES), a study that attempts to measure our health and establish the probable causes for disease. In a study conducted by the Centers for Disease Control (CDC) in 2003, it was shown that one out of six women of childbearing age had toxic levels of mercury in their bodies. It is a widely accepted fact that during pregnancy a vast amount of nutrients are diverted from the mother to support the growth of the baby. It was previously thought that the mother's placenta filtered out harmful substances, providing a barrier between toxic exposure to the mother and similar exposure to the baby. Now we know that, along with life-supporting nutrition, potentially harmful substances are transferred from mother to baby. At the 2004 U.S. Environmental Protection Agency's National Forum on Contaminants in Fish, EPA biochemist Kathryn R. Mahaffey reported that researchers had conclusively shown mercury levels in umbilical cord blood are typically 70 percent higher than levels in the mother's blood. It becomes painfully clear that if one out of every six women giving birth in our country has toxic levels of mercury, some, if not most, of that mercury is being shunted to the developing baby, especially to its developing brain.

Furthermore, according to the Autism A.L.A.R.M. report released in early 2004 by the U.S. Department of Health and Human Services, the Centers for Disease Control, and the American Academy of Pediatrics, one of out every six children born in the United States suffers from some type of developmental disorder and/or behavioral problem. Because this statistic mirrors the number of women with mercury toxicity, many medical professionals are concerned about a correlation between the two. Virtually all neurological issues affecting children after birth—including but not limited to attention deficit disorder (ADD), attention deficit hyperactivity disorder (ADHD), pervasive developmental disorders (PDD), and autism spectrum disorders (ASD)—are associated with some level of mercury in their bodies.

On July 14, 2005, a well-respected, privately funded, nonprofit research organization known as the Environmental Working Group (EWG) released a report titled "Body Burden: The Pollution in Newborns." The EWG tested umbilical cord blood from newborn babies for 413 industrial chemicals, pollutants, and pesticides, and found 287 of these substances present in the samples obtained. Mercury was detected in all samples, and of the 287 substances found, 180 are known to "cause cancer in humans or animals, 217 are toxic to the brain and nervous system, and 208 are known to cause birth defects or abnormal development in animal tests." The summary of this report noted the following:

> . . . some of the umbilical cord blood collected by the Red Cross after the cord was cut harbored pesticides, consumer product ingredients, and wastes from burning coal, gasoline, and garbage. The dangers of pre- or postnatal exposure to this complex mixture of carcinogens, developmental toxins, and neurotoxins have never been studied.
>
> Chemical exposures in the womb or during infancy can be dramatically more harmful than exposures later in life. Substantial scientific evidence demonstrates that children face amplified risks from their body burden of pollution; the findings are particularly strong for many of the chemicals found in this study, including mercury, PCBs, and dioxins. Children's vulnerability derives from both rapid development and incomplete defense systems:
>
> - A developing child's chemical exposures are greater pound for pound than those of adults.
> - An immature, porous blood-brain barrier allows greater chemical exposures to the developing brain.
> - Children have lower levels of some chemical-binding proteins, allowing more of a chemical to reach "target organs."

- A baby's organs and systems are rapidly developing, and thus are often more vulnerable to damage from chemical exposure.
- Systems that detoxify and excrete industrial chemicals are not fully developed.
- The longer future life span of a child compared to an adult allows more time for adverse effects to arise.

A developing baby depends on adults for protection, nutrition, and, ultimately, survival. As a society we have a responsibility to ensure that babies do not enter this world pre-polluted, with 200 industrial chemicals in their blood.

Mercury and Autism

Children with autism (mercury toxicity) have many resulting imbalances in their systems, such as significant allergies, opportunistic infections, hormonal imbalances, gastrointestinal disorders, immune dysfunctions, and nutritional deficiencies. However, these are what I refer to as the "fires" of autism. All these, and other fires of autism, result from one major "spark": mercury! Successfully addressing these fires will provide temporary improvement, but until the spark (mercury) that constantly reignites these fires has definitively been eliminated, any improvement will be short lived at best.

We've seen that children diagnosed with autism suffer from acute mercury toxicity due to exposure through their mothers before they are born and early on in life from vaccinations. Adults diagnosed with Alzheimer's, on the other hand, suffer from chronic, insidious mercury toxicity from exposure over the years from amalgam in their teeth, the inhalation of mercury vapors and by-products of fossil fuel combustion, and diet, among others. By addressing and eliminating the mercury spark, both autism and Alzheimer's become far easier to manage and the improvements from treatment become easier to maintain. In fact, along with some supportive therapies, these illnesses can be fully and permanently reversed if appropriately treated. This is *not* theory. It has been clinically validated on a repetitive basis and the evidence is irrefutable.

The reason some individuals suffer severe damage from mercury when others don't is due to factors such as biological individuality and genetic predisposition. In addition, how the individual was exposed—whether by inhalation, digestion, injection, or skin exposure—makes an enormous difference. It also matters what type of mercury exposure the individual received—organic or inorganic mercury—and if organic, whether it was ethyl mercury or methyl mercury.

Other factors include the following:

- The frequency of exposure to the source of toxicity.
- Whether there was exposure from the mother before birth.
- Whether the mother was inoculated or had RhoGAM either during pregnancy or prior to conception.

- The number of vaccine administrations and over what period of time.
- Exposure through diet.
- The proximity to industrial sites and exposure to fossil fuel pollution.

As you can see, there are many variables that can lead to autism, but the treatment is essentially the same. The only difference is how long treatment needs to extend. The basis for how we treat children diagnosed with autism was determined by my clinical observation that some children were unable to detoxify the mercury in their bodies as well as other children. The only solution for children who cannot eliminate mercury on their own is to administer effective treatments for removing the mercury, while repairing and enhancing their immune systems.

My Personal Experience with Autism

On January 25, 1999, my son Abid Azam Ali Buttar was born. By the time he was fourteen or fifteen months old, he was already saying "abu" (which means father in Arabic) and a few other words, such as "bye-bye." But by the age of eighteen months, my son had not only failed to progress in his ability to speak, but had also lost the few words he had been saying. As he grew older, I began to worry more and more that he was suffering from a developmental delay. He exhibited the same characteristics noticed by many parents with children who have developmental delays: stemming (self-stimulation that includes repetitive actions, movements, or sounds), walking on tiptoes, and lack of eye contact. Sometimes I would call to him, but his lack of response would convince me there must be something wrong with his hearing. Certain sounds would make him cringe, and he would put his hands over his ears to block the obvious discomfort he was experiencing. He would spend hours watching the oscillation of a fan. But through all this, when he would make eye contact with me, his eyes would say, "I know you can do it, Dad."

The oceans of tears that I cried and the hours that I spent trying to determine what was happening to my son are no different from what any other parent in the same situation experiences. The only difference was that I was one of approximately 190 doctors in the United States who was board certified in clinical metal toxicology. If my son's problem was metal related, I should know how to fix it. I tested and retested him, and tested him again, searching for mercury. But the older he became, the more obvious it was that my son was not developing as he should; that was the only thing I knew for certain. From the time Abie lost his speech, at around eighteen months of age, until he was three years old, he had absolutely no verbal communication except for the one syllable that he would utter on a repetitive basis: "deh."

While desperately searching for the cause of the same ailment that had afflicted so many of my own patients, I was invited to present a lecture. This offered me an opportunity to discuss my son's situation with Boyd Haley, chairman of the department of chemistry at the University of Kentucky. That meeting led to a discussion about a study that at that time had not yet been published, which turned out to be key to our development of a protocol for treating children with autism, autism-like spectrum disorder, and pervasive developmental delay. My son was the first child who went through this protocol once it had been safety established.

In the late 1990s, Dr. Haley had teamed up with two other researchers, A. S. Holmes and M. F. Blaxill, to do a study assessing the level of mercury measured in the hair of forty-five normally developing children versus ninety-four children with neurodevelopmental delays diagnosed as autism. The finding showed that the autistic children had 0.47 parts per million of mercury in their hair, and the normally developing children had 3.63 parts per million, more that seven times the same level of mercury as the autistic children. Opponents of Dr. Holmes's study (and his theory of mercury neurodegeneration) insisted that mercury had nothing to do with autism or any other neurodegenerative condition. However, they completely missed the point of the study. The conclusion of the study is obvious, and in part, is reproduced below:

> The reduced levels of mercury in the first baby haircut of autistic infants raise clear questions about the detoxification capacity of a subset of infants. Despite hair levels suggesting low exposure, these infants had measured exposures at least equal to the control population, suggesting that the control infants were able to eliminate mercury more effectively. In the case of autistic infants, those in our sample were exposed to higher levels of mercury during gestation, through dental amalgams or Rho D immunoglobulin injections in the mother. The addition of multiple postnatal exposures to mercury in childhood vaccines would have more severe consequences in infants whose detoxification capacity is reduced or who may be closer to a dangerous threshold of exposure. In the case of the control infants, mercury hair levels were strongly affected by exposure levels, suggesting that detoxification and excretion played an important role in ensuring normal development in children with elevated toxic exposure relative to their peers. If reduced overall mercury elimination is related to hair elimination, then autistic infants will retain significantly higher levels of mercury in their tissues, including the brain, than normal infants. In light of the biological plausibility of mercury's role in neurodevelopmental disorders, our study provides further insight into one possible mechanism by which early mercury exposures could increase the risk of autism.

These findings were published in the *International Journal of Toxicology* in 2003. Understanding these findings, along with my clinical experience, led me to the conclusion that a more aggressive method of treatment was necessary than the use of DMSA (a chelating agent used to eliminate mercury and other heavy metals) and unsuccessful methods I had used to try to document high levels of mercury in my son. After six tests to find mercury in his system (including three tests using DMPS, another chelating agent), we discovered his mercury level was over 400 percent that of safe levels. It is important to note that this level was only indicative of what we were able to "elicit or sequester" out of him. His actual levels were far greater.

I started Abie's treatments on his third birthday, using a rudimentary version of the current TD-DMPS (DMPS in a transdermal base) that my partner Dean Viktora and I had experimented with a few years previously. By the time Abie was about three and a half, five months after initiating treatment with TD-DMPS, my son started to speak, progressing so rapidly that his speech therapist commented that she'd never seen such rapid progress in a child before. Today, at the age of five, Abie's development is far ahead of his peers, having learned prayers in a second language, doing large mathematical calculations in his head, playing chess, and reading simple three- and four-letter words. His attention span and focus were sufficiently advanced to the point of being accepted as the youngest child into a martial arts academy when he was only four. His vocabulary is as extensive as any ten-year-old's, and his sense of humor, power to reason, and ability to understand detailed and complex concepts constantly amaze me.

Abie's recovery was the basis for our study analyzing the extraordinary results obtained in his treatment and the subsequent treatment of thirty-one other children in the same manner. These patients had diagnoses of autism, autism-like spectrum disorder, and pervasive developmental delay. In order to be included in the study, each child received an independent diagnosis of these conditions from a neurologist or pediatrician. Also, we required the agreement of their parents to try treatment using TD-DMPS; those patients whose parents did not wish them to be treated with the TD-DMPS were not included. Some of the older children (those over the age of eight) received DMPS intravenously and were not included in this study. However, it's important to note how willing parents were to get successful treatment for their children.

All thirty-one children were tested for metal toxicity every two months for a year and then every four months after that, using urine metal toxicity and essential minerals, hair metal toxicity and essential minerals, red blood cell metal toxicity, and fecal metal toxicity. In the initial test results, the children in the study showed little or no level of mercury. Subsequent tests showed significantly higher levels of mercury as treatment continued, approximately a 350 percent increase after two months. (Quite often mercury level tests will measure low or show no mercury in the beginning of chelation therapy. It is believed that the reason children exhibit autistic symptoms is because their bodies cannot detox from the heavy metals, and they require several sessions of chelation therapy to get the mercury moving out. Therefore, as treatment continues, higher levels of mercury begin to be released and the autistic symptoms start to reverse. For more information on this study, please visit www.drbuttar.com/articles.)

The more mercury that was eliminated, the more noticeable were the clinical improvements and the more dramatic the change in the children's behavior. Several children who had no prior history of speech started to speak at the age of six or seven, sometimes in full sentences. The children also exhibited substantially improved behavior: the reduction and eventual cessation of all stemming behavior; the return of full eye contact; and rapid potty training, sometimes in children who were five or six but had never been successfully potty trained. Additional findings reported by parents included an increase in the rate of physical growth as well as improvement in the ability to follow instructions, increased affection and social interaction with siblings and/or other children, active seeking of interaction with others, appropriate social responses, and a rapid acceleration of verbal skills. The results for many of these children were documented on video, and other physicians using this type of treatment have been able to reproduce the same results successfully.

DMPS (dimercaptopropane–1 sulfonate) is primarily mercury and arsenic. (Chelators are organic chemicals that bond with and remove free metal ions.) Parents and professionals should understand that the use of DMPS has its pitfalls as well as advantages. When taken orally, 50–55 percent of DMPS is normally absorbed in the digestive tract. But because children with autism often have compromised gastrointestinal function, there is decreased absorption of oral DMPS. Most of the children who took oral DMPS continuously for more than one week complained of abdominal pain, cramping, and other digestive distress. We tried oral DMPS for almost six weeks before eliminating it as a possible treatment method. Intravenous DMPS was not an option for young children, although it's the method I prefer and what I use in my clinical practice for my adult patients with mercury toxicity. All the children in the study were also monitored for kidney function and mineral depletion.

The key to success with this study was the constant and continuous "pull" of mercury that resulted from providing doses of DMPS every other day. We used transdermal DMPS (TD-DMPS), which is DMPS conjugated with a number of amino acids, in a base that includes essential fatty acids. Frequent dosing is one of the most important components of treatment with TD-DMPS. Although DMPS is very unstable when exposed to air, this and many other issues with it have been resolved over the last few years, with the final result now pending patent. In addition, various amino acids and glutathione have been added to TD-DMPS to make it more effective.

Even though there are a number of substances that successfully remove mercury from someone suffering from mercury toxicity, the most important aspect of the elimination process is the removal of the source of mercury. Once this has been done, detoxification can begin.

There has been extensive research in both safety and effectiveness of DMPS in the fifty years of its existence, and it is now considered to be the most effective therapy for the treatment of mercury toxicity. DMPS is very safe when used properly. Side effects are very rare but may include allergic reactions, such as skin rashes. It is most important to monitor intake and also supplement with appropriate doses of zinc and copper, as these minerals are bound readily by DMPS in the same way as DMPS binds mercury. Supplementation should be done prior to the commencement of any DMPS treatment regimen and periodically through-out the process.

Currently, there are a number of different professional medical organizations that teach physicians the appropriate methods of effectively chelating toxic met-als, such as the International College of Integrative Medicine, American College for Advancement of Medicine, and Integrative Therapeutics in Anti-Aging. These organizations periodically conduct workshops on mercury toxicity, with specific emphasis on both basic scientific knowledge and clinical evaluation and treatment.

With the increased concern about mercury toxicity as an environmental health threat, and in recognition of the need to increase basic scientific research and clinical treatment of heavy metal toxicity, the American Board of Clinical Metal Toxicology (ABCMT) was recently formed as an evolution of the American Board of Chelation Therapy. This board will greatly expand the educational opportuni-ties for physicians interested in this health problem, and will offer them certification in the competency and proficiency in the clinical removal of heavy metal toxic-ity. As a result of the work of these organizations, a general protocol for the use of DMPS has been established that most certified physicians follow.

DMSA is now thought to be potentially harmful if used in patients with exces-sively high levels of mercury. Therefore, DMSA is recommended only for use late in the mercury elimination process, after the peripheral tissue load of mer-cury has been reduced by DMPS. In our observations, DMSA did not show efficacy in removing mercury or in clinical improvement in children diagnosed with autism or PDD. The yield of DMPS compared to DMSA for removal of mercury in this example was ten to one.

In our clinical experience, the safest and only effective method that has result-ed in the consistent, slow removal of mercury resulting in the elimination of this "spark" in the pediatric population is the TD-DMPS, which was originally for-mulated only for the purposes of treating my son's developmental delay. Since its implementation, we have now successfully treated scores of patients, many of whom have completely recovered and all of whom have improved since the imple-mentation of this treatment. These results have been duplicated by other physicians involved with the care of patients with neurodegenerative disease processes.

Summary

The underlying common denominator in chronic neurodegenerative disease seems to be either decreasing vascular supply (less blood to the brain) or accumulation of heavy metals, specifically mercury. The inability of an individ-ual to eliminate toxic metals, especially mercury, is directly related to the level of neurodegeneration experienced. In the young patient population suffering from autism or pervasive developmental delay, vascular supply is not an issue. The under-lying pathology of children with autism and the geriatric population with Alzheimer's is of the same cause, specifically mercury toxicity.

Both patient populations suffer from the inability to excrete mercury as a result of a genetic predisposition resulting from various factors. If these patient populations inhabited a completely mercury-free environment, they would not have the problems associated with autism or Alzheimer's. When the mercury is successfully removed from their systems, these individuals begin to significantly improve, as evidenced by steady improvement in cognitive function.

Mercury is the "spark" that causes the "fires" of autism as well as many other neurodegenerative diseases, including PDD, ADD, ADHD, and Alzheimer's. Autism is the result of high mercury exposure early in life, versus Alzheimer's where there is a chronic accumulation of mercury over a lifetime. A doctor can treat *all* the "fires," but until the "spark" is removed, there is minimal hope of complete recovery, with most realized improvements being transient at best. Mercury is the underlying common denominator of all the problems from which these children suffer. And the only solution for them is to effectively remove the mercury while repairing and enhancing the damaged elimination and detoxification pathways. Addressing the GI tract at the same time is vital if the goal of treatment is to achieve permanent recovery.

Once the process of mercury removal has been effectively initiated, the source of damage is curtailed and full recovery becomes possible. Complete recovery can then be attained and further enhanced by utilizing various additional essential therapies like nutrition. It is my hope and prayer, along with the hopes and prayers of all clinicians who are cognizant of these facts, that the U.S. Congress will act quickly and decisively and put an end to this legalized and tolerated mass modern genocide by outlawing the use of mercury-based preservatives in all childhood and adult vaccines.

—*Rashid A. Buttar, DO, FAAPM, FACAM, FAAIM*

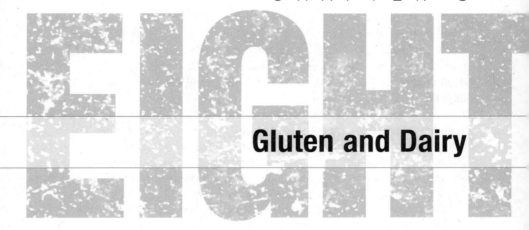

Gluten and Dairy

HIDDEN TOXINS AND HOW THEY CONTRIBUTE TO DIGESTIVE DISORDERS

Allergies to wheat and/or gluten and dairy products are surprisingly common among children and adults suffering from the symptoms of ADHD. Removing the foods that cause the allergic reaction can have enormous beneficial results.

"Bread is the staff of life" is a common refrain I hear from my clients who are asked to reduce or remove bread from their diets. Bread and grains are so highly valued worldwide that the word "bread" is sometimes used to refer to food in general, as in the phrase "breaking bread." Most every culture believes that bread and grains should occupy the center of a nutritious diet. Unfortunately, this belief could not be further from the truth; in fact, grain foods are likely partially at fault for many chronic diseases that affect society. While it is true that a diet high in grains will prevent someone from starving to death, it will not allow him or her to maintain or achieve good health.

Anthropological evidence shows that grains have only been a part of the human diet for about twelve thousand years, originating in the Middle East, where populations were among the first to farm grains. Among Aboriginal and American Indian populations, grains have been consumed for only a few hundred years. In the grand scheme of things, this is a very short period of time, particularly when we consider that this is the amount of time the complex human body has had to adapt to this new food. Grains were unlike any source of nutrition that we had been eating up until that point—mainly the vegetables, fruits, nuts, and meats that we had evolved to eat over the course of many millions of years. Therefore, it is not surprising that so many of us have difficulty properly digesting them.

Recent discoveries using DNA analysis have shown that as humans began farming grains their stature changed dramatically. In fact, over the course of only a few generations, our agricultural ancestors decreased in height by five to six inches while their head circumference, a marker correlated with brain size, decreased by 11 percent. Amazingly, this happened after only a few generations of eating a diet high in grains.

To further exacerbate the negative effects that grains have on our bodies, our agricultural practices are constantly forcing grains to evolve further. This usually involves creating grains with higher and higher protein content to allow them to reproduce more quickly and in harsher climates. When we change the nutrient profiles of these foods, our bodies are further taxed in their effort to fully adapt to them and learn how to use them properly.

Digestion is a somewhat complex process that begins with the chewing of food and continues when the food is chemically broken down by specific digestive enzymes. The process ends when the food is fully broken down and absorbed through the gastrointestinal wall into the bloodstream. Only when these processes are completed can we use the nutrients in our foods to fuel our bodies and minds.

Gluten, the protein in wheat and related grains (including barley, rye, oats, spelt, kamut, and triticale), is particularly difficult to fully digest. Gluten is held together by sulfide bonds, which are very difficult to break. For this reason, gluten is only ever partially digested. Moreover, gluten-containing grains contain enzyme inhibitors, which interfere with protein breakdown, further reducing the body's ability to digest these grains properly. Eating gluten-containing foods frequently may exhaust the body's enzyme supplies, exacerbating poor digestion.

Dairy products, particularly homogenized dairy products, are also difficult for many people to digest because of the substances created during this process. Because proteins in gluten-containing grains and dairy products are not fully broken down, they wreak havoc on the digestive system. Not only are the nutrients from these foods not absorbed, but gluten-containing grains and dairy products also have other more detrimental and long-lasting effects.

The most devastating effects of gluten and dairy malabsorption are found within the immune system. Approximately 60 percent of our immune system resides in our gastrointestinal tract. This portion of our immune system is called gut-associated lymphoid tissue (GALT), and it serves as our first defense against an attack on our body. This tissue launches the first assault against the common cold, kills bacteria that finds its way into our food, and combats toxins from our environment. We are bombarded by bacteria, viruses, chemicals, and other antigens, but a healthy gastrointestinal tract fights these predators without us even knowing it. We only feel the effects of these toxins if they make it past this first defense. For this reason, the health of our gastrointestinal tract is paramount to overall good health.

When we consume a diet containing gluten and dairy, we are directly contributing to poor gastrointestinal health due to the poor digestion of these foods. When gluten and dairy proteins aren't broken down as a result of inadequate enzymes, enzyme inhibitors, or other factors, these proteins remain in the gastrointestinal tract as large particles. This wouldn't be so bad if these particles were excreted. Instead, GALT gets involved and attempts to determine what these larger proteins are. Since it cannot properly categorize these particles, it treats them as predators, or toxins, and launches an immune attack against them.

The immune attack process results in irritation of the gastrointestinal tract. The tissues get inflamed in the same way that the mucous membranes of your nose get inflamed when you have a cold or flu. In addition, they release a protective mucous layer to prevent absorption of the toxin, similar to how your nose runs when you have a cold. This process wouldn't be problematic if it only occurred a few times a year, like a cold or flu; when it occurs very regularly, however, it becomes troublesome.

The average American eats at least one, and often many more, gluten- or dairy-containing foods every day; it is estimated that 19 percent of the American diet is composed of gluten-containing foods. That means this process is affecting most Americans to one degree or another almost every day. When your gastrointestinal tract is in a constant state of inflammation, you develop a condition called leaky gut syndrome. This condition is very common in children with ADD/ADHD, autism, allergies, chemical sensitivities, and many chronic illnesses.

Leaky gut is characterized as a combination of both underabsorption and overabsorption within the gastrointestinal tract. When the gut becomes inflamed as a result of an immune attack, it becomes more permeable and less able to properly mediate the passage of particles into the bloodstream. As a result, food particles that have not been fully broken down are allowed to pass out of the intestine and into the bloodstream at points of inflammation. In addition, increased mucus within the gut blocks the absorption of digested food particles where the mucus is present.

While it may seem counterintuitive that a leaky gut allows large particles into the bloodstream and blocks small particles, the effects can be illustrated by one of the common diagnostic tests for this condition. Leaky gut syndrome is often diagnosed by administering a lactulose-mannitol test. During this test, you drink a solution containing mannitol and lactulose and then collect your urine over a period of time. Mannitol is made up of small molecules that should be very easily absorbed from the intestinal tract and excreted in urine, while lactulose is made up of larger molecules that are not normally absorbed and, as a result, are excreted in feces. For a person with a healthy gastrointestinal tract, the amount of mannitol in the urine should be high and lactulose should be very low or nonexistent. With leaky gut syndrome, the amount of lactulose in the urine is much higher, while mannitol levels can vary depending on the severity of the case. Thus large, poorly absorbed molecules are absorbed, and depending on the severity of mucus production, small, easily absorbed molecules are not absorbed. This pattern extends to all substances that enter the gastrointestinal tract.

When undigested food particles and other foreign substances are allowed to enter the bloodstream, they can trigger other immune responses that affect the entire body, not just the gut. This leads to hypersensitivity to foods, the environment, and normally benign substances.

Cerebral allergies are a typical consequence of this immune response, and wheat and milk are the most common culprits. Cerebral allergies are the basis of allergy-addiction cycles, where the body craves certain allergens to avoid withdrawal symptoms. With leaky gut syndrome, certain antigens or antigen-antibody complexes enter the bloodstream and then cross the blood-brain barrier and negatively affect brain health. Common symptoms include anxiety, irritability, aggression, and even psychotic episodes. This phenomenon is very common in children because they often eat very limited diets with little variety.

The gastrointestinal tract not only works to break down food and allow its absorption, it also serves as the body's first barrier against attacks from foreign molecules. It protects against bacteria, viruses, fungi, chemicals, heavy metals, and any other particles that might find their way into your body via the GI tract. With increased gastrointestinal permeability, these particles are more readily absorbed. This can lead to chronic bacterial, viral, and fungal infections; heavy metal poisoning; and chemical sensitivities, among other health problems. Some of these toxins are even able to cross the blood-brain barrier and wreak havoc within the central nervous system. This is particularly noteworthy in the case of heavy metal poisoning because of the extensive harm that heavy metals can have on the nervous system.

Any toxin that enters the body, and many endogenous chemicals (like hormones and inflammation complexes) made within the body, need to be detoxified before they can be safely excreted. This detoxification occurs primarily within the liver and mucous membranes, and relies upon certain enzymes, nutrients, and biochemical processes, collectively referred to as detoxification pathways. The body's ability to eliminate these toxins and endogenous chemicals is limited by its supply of the necessary enzymes and nutrients. Therefore, when the toxin level exceeds the capacity of the detoxification pathways, toxins enter into the bloodstream, accumulate, and damage the body. This phenomenon is often referred to as the "rain barrel effect," where the body is doing just fine as toxins accumulate, but once they completely fill the "rain barrel" and begin to flow over, health problems ensue. Once your "rain barrel" is full, your detoxification pathways are at their limit, and toxins are now able to wreak havoc on your body.

With leaky gut syndrome, not only do greater levels of toxins enter the bloodstream, but along with them high levels of inflammatory immune complexes are delivered to the liver. This stresses the body's detoxification pathways further, allowing an even greater number of toxins into the bloodstream. The likelihood of these toxins entering the brain and nervous system increases greatly at this point, and the body's ability to detoxify is simultaneously diminished due to the increased toxic load on the liver. This vicious cycle of accumulating toxins creates an overall decrease in health.

Chronic infections, elevated heavy metal levels, and chemical sensitivities often coexist in cases of ADD and ADHD. The symptoms of ADD and ADHD often reverse when these other conditions are removed. Thus, addressing these toxins is paramount to healing, and the first step is addressing the increased permeability of the gastrointestinal tract and stopping these antigens from being reintroduced into the body. In fact, many of my clients are never able to fully reverse their mercury, lead, and other heavy metal toxicity until they first heal their leaky gut; this frequently happens despite their use of heavy metal chelation with DMSA and other chelating agents. In other clients, I have seen a reversal of heavy metal levels by merely healing the gut without chelation therapy.

Thankfully, leaky gut syndrome is reversible. The process of reversal involves allowing the gut to heal so that it can return to normal functioning. This usually requires several steps and can take months, but the results are quite amazing.

The first step always involves removing the offending foods from the diet. For most of my clients that means avoiding all gluten-containing foods and usually avoiding dairy products as well. This stops the immune attack that begins in the gut and allows the GI tract to heal. The process of healing can be monitored with follow-up lactulose-mannitol tests showing a return to healthy levels. When clients watch their progress, it often provides them with the necessary motivation to continue with this step, which is by far the most difficult. When working with children, it is especially important to find replacements for the foods that are being removed from their diets. Fortunately, so many people are avoiding these foods these days that alternatives can be found at most natural food stores. Rice-based breads and pastas serve as excellent substitutes for their gluten-containing counterparts, and nut-based milks and cheeses, also available at most natural food stores, are good replacements for similar dairy products. Soymilk and soy-based cheeses are another option, but in my experience children generally prefer the taste and texture of the nut-based alternatives.

Beyond removing the offending foods, taking full-spectrum digestive enzymes with each meal can be quite beneficial, as they help with the breakdown of all foods. Each enzyme targets a particular food type and assists in its breakdown. For example, amylase digests amylose, a type of carbohydrate, but it does not digest lactose, a different type of carbohydrate, nor does it digest lipids or proteins. Full-spectrum digestive enzymes contain protein-digesting enzymes like papain and various proteases, along with the fat-digesting enzyme lipase, and a number of carbohydrate-digesting enzymes like amylase and invertase. These enzymes provide additional digestive assistance and increase the likelihood that your food will be in the appropriately digested state by the time it is absorbed. In addition to augmenting your naturally occurring enzymes, full-spectrum digestive enzymes provide enzymes that your body may not make or that you do not make enough of. This step alone can have a profound, positive effect on digestion and the reversal of leaky gut syndrome.

The next step I recommend is adding omega-3 fatty acids, usually from fish oils, but vegetarian sources are quite acceptable as well. These oils help reduce inflammation by halting the cascade of arachidonic acid. By reducing inflammation in this manner, intestinal healing will progress more quickly. It is important to note that this step also has a profound effect on ADD and ADHD in general. By removing inflammation within the brain and nervous system, the symptoms of ADD and ADHD can be significantly reduced.

The final step I recommend in healing the gut is the use of probiotics, which help increase the amount of beneficial bacteria and yeast in the intestinal tract. These microbes further help break down your food and also prevent the colonization of unfriendly bacteria that contribute to poor gastrointestinal health. Because both friendly and unfriendly microbes use the same food sources, a high level of friendly bacteria in the gut can prevent unfriendly bacteria from colonizing by essentially starving them of their food source. It is important to note that the primary food source for these microbes is sugar. Thus, if the diet is high in sugar, both the friendly and unfriendly microbes will feast and flourish. Therefore, to have the greatest positive effect on your gastrointestinal flora, you should greatly limit sugar consumption and reduce carbohydrate consumption in general, as carbohydrates are easily broken down into sugars during digestion. Most children with ADHD have been found to have abnormal cortisol rhythms, a condition that is frequently associated with poor carbohydrate metabolism, resulting in an even greater need to limit sugar intake.

While leaky gut syndrome is definitely one of the most profoundly negative outcomes of a diet that includes gluten and dairy products, it is not the only consequence. In addition to promoting a leaky gut, gluten and dairy products are high in certain proteins called lectins, which adversely affect the nervous system.

Lectins are proteins that bind to carbohydrates, usually on cell membranes. The cell membrane is a site of heavy activity, as this is where the cell determines whether or not a molecule can enter. When this activity is compromised, the cell no longer functions properly. Lectins bind to cell membranes and disrupt this activity; depending on the degree of dysfunction that is caused, it could lead to cell death.

This is particularly noteworthy for the cells of the nervous system, as their primary activity is to create a synaptic potential (also called nerve cell firings). All information within the nervous system is transmitted via a carefully orchestrated series of synaptic potentials. A synaptic potential is only allowed to occur if certain channels on the cell membrane are able to properly open and close, allowing electrolytes, like calcium and potassium, to cross the cell membrane and create an electrochemical charge. When the cell membrane is not working properly, this electrochemical charge does not occur appropriately. This could mean that the nerve cells fire when they shouldn't or don't fire when they should. In either case, the nervous system is compromised, resulting in a variety of possible neurological dysfunctions, including ADD and ADHD.

Gluten and dairy products are both high in the lectins that have been directly implicated in ADD and ADHD. It is also worth mentioning that these effects are seen with a greater regularity in people consuming dairy products from grain-fed cattle rather than grass-fed cattle.

When looking at the big picture and seeing how gluten and dairy products negatively affect the body and mind in so many disparate ways, it seems like an easy decision to remove these foods from our diets. Based on the results I have seen in my practice, I can assure you that, despite any challenges you might face, it is a very worthwhile endeavor. Fortunately, we live in a time when gluten-free and dairy-free substitutes for almost any food are readily available at your local natural food store. Even if ADD or ADHD affects only your child, you may find that when you remove these foods from your diet along with your child's diet, any symptoms that you may be experiencing will be reduced as well. Time and again I have seen parents notice a reduction in their own respiratory allergies, arthritis, headaches, insomnia, depression, and many other symptoms just by removing these foods. Gluten-containing grains and dairy products are foods that we could all benefit from avoiding.

—Trisha Ann Ochoa, CHN

IV

Balancing the Brain and Body

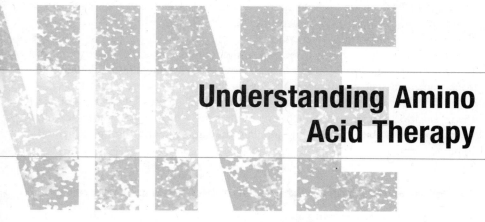

Understanding Amino Acid Therapy

A NATURAL APPROACH TO BALANCING YOUR CHILD'S BRAIN

Balancing your child's brain is an important part of optimizing his or her life, and it often helps to solve the symptoms of ADHD. When your child's brain is balanced, remarkable improvement and success occurs in the ability to handle situations that previously caused distress. The child begins interacting appropriately with family and in social situations and excels academically, problematic behaviors subside, and neurological gaps lessen. Amino acid therapy is an important piece of the puzzle when solving behavioral and emotional issues through a scientific and natural approach.

The Case of Charlie

Charlie is a charismatic ten-year-old boy with a good sense of humor. He likes swimming, video games, and science. He is often described as the class clown, and teachers report that he talks too much in class. Charlie was diagnosed with attention deficit hyperactivity disorder, which makes it difficult for him to remain calm, complete tasks, and pay attention. Additionally, it's difficult for him to succeed academically, which has decreased his self-esteem and increased his frustration. His distractibility is evident at home and has been for years. His mother reports that she's constantly reminding him to do things, stating that homework and chores are a nightmare and take hours to complete. Charlie becomes frustrated easily and often has meltdowns when trying to complete the simplest tasks.

After trying stimulant medications, Charlie's parents felt discouraged and fearful for Charlie's and the family's future. His cheerful demeanor was replaced with anger, and Charlie soon became aggressive, noncompliant, and withdrawn. His weight plummeted, and his anxiety manifested into obsessive thoughts to the point that he was unable to fall asleep at night.

This experience not only affected Charlie, but also his entire family's functioning. Their home turned from a safe and loving environment into a chaotic war zone, causing disharmony among all. His parents could no longer handle the distress of Charlie's ADHD and the adverse affects of his medications. They stopped the medication regimen and sought out another route. With the help of a trained practitioner, they began adjusting his neurotransmitter levels through a natural approach: amino acid therapy.

Overview of Amino Acids and Neurotransmitters

As you may recall from your middle school biology class, amino acids are the building blocks of life and the precursors to our neurotransmitters. Neurotransmitters are the brain chemicals that communicate information throughout our brain and body. They also affect our mood, sleep, concentration, and weight, and can cause adverse symptoms when they are out of balance, as seen with Charlie.

Neurotransmitter levels can be depleted many ways. It is estimated that 86 percent of Americans have suboptimal neurotransmitter levels. Personalized amino acid therapy is the use of supplemental amino acids to help balance brain chemicals (neurotransmitters) and other aspects of the physiology. For this type of treatment to be most effective, it should include a specialized urine test that provides a reliable means of measuring excretory values for neurotransmitters. The most effective patient outcomes result from specific laboratory assessments developed in Germany utilizing their normative data. From those findings, an individualized protocol of amino acid supplementation is devised to improve the quantity and ratios of neurotransmitters in the brain. Today there are seven major neurotransmitters that are tested. They are the most empirically valid and are the precursors to other, lower-chain amino acids.

Neurotransmitters fall into two categories: inhibitory and excitatory. Ideally, they should be balanced. However, the neurotransmitters of many children (and adults) are not. Genetics, stress, nutrition, early childhood experiences, traumas, neglect, and abuse all play a part in our neurotransmitter makeup.

Excitatory neurotransmitters are not necessarily exciting; they are what stimulate the brain. These neurotransmitters, which are tested through urine analysis, are dopamine, norepinephrine, epinephrine, and glutamate. When the excitatory side is too high, problems start to occur, such as disrupted sleep, focus difficulties, and meltdowns.

Inhibitory neurotransmitters are those that calm the brain and help balance one's mood. They are easily depleted when excitatory neurotransmitters are overactive. Inhibitory neurotransmitters include serotonin, dopamine (mildly inhibitory), and GABA. It's difficult to correct mood imbalances with behavior methods alone. Even with the best intentions, a child may not be able to change his behavior because of his brain chemistry profile; it may be beyond his capacity. Here's a brief overview of what each neurotransmitter does and how it plays a role in your child's mental health and behavior:

- **Dopamine** is an inhibitory and excitatory neurotransmitter; it is responsible for addictive behaviors, focus and memory issues, and disruption in motivation and drive. We see compulsive tendencies and obsessive behaviors in many children with disrupted dopamine. When dopamine is extremely elevated there's an inability to control behaviors; impulsivity and aggressive behaviors in children become more pervasive. When dopamine is low, ADD or focus issues are typically present.

- **Epinephrine** is also responsible for "fight or flight" response in accordance with norepinephrine. This excitatory neurotransmitter response is responsible for energy, depression, cognitive function, hyperactivity, stress, ADHD symptoms, and insomnia.

- **GABA** is an inhibitory neurotransmitter responsible for calming the brain. When it is too high or low, children experience sleeplessness or disrupted sleep, overactivity, inability to calm oneself, quickness to respond, and impulsive behavior. Regulation of GABA is an intrinsic part in resolving sleep-cycle issues and lowering overactive excitatory neurotransmitters.

- **Glutamate** is an excitatory neurotransmitter. When it is out of balance, it is responsible for agitation, sleeplessness, focus issues, and depression. These symptoms can be reduced when the child's brain gets more inhibitory support, which helps to suppress the expression of these behaviors.

- **Serotonin** is an inhibitory neurotransmitter generally referred to as the "feel good neurotransmitter" and is involved in regulating one's mood. When serotonin is out of balance, we tend to see disturbances in mood, low self-esteem, disruption in sleep, agitation, carbohydrate craving, high anxiety, and high stress.

- **Norepinephrine** is an excitatory neurotransmitter; when it is overactive or underactive, children act out in negative behaviors. Energy, drive, stimulation, "fight or flight" response, insomnia, anxiety, and mood are affected when this neutrotransmitter is out of balance. Norepinephrine is responsible for epinephrine levels, and generally when we see low or high levels of one, the other is affected similarly. With kids who are hyperactive or unable to focus, this neurotransmitter is usually fairly high and is reflected in their inability to control behavior, soothe themselves, or pay attention.

The results of Charlie's neurotransmitter levels showed that his inhibitory levels were extremely depleted, making his excitatory levels pervasive, and thus creating his lack of control and attention. This was evident in his behavior; he was unable to calm himself down, pay attention, or stay on task because of this chemical imbalance. He lacked the inhibitory support, which exacerbated the symptoms of his ADHD. Stimulant medications for ADD/ADHD cause dopamine to be pushed into the synapse so that focus is improved. Unfortunately, stimulating dopamine consistently can cause depletion over time. Charlie's excitatory level was very high, making it nearly impossible for him to calm down and focus. His test results indicated that he was chemically unable to focus; he didn't have a choice.

Charlie began taking amino acid supplements that provided him with the "food" his brain so desperately needed to synthesize neurotransmitters. Specific amino acid ratios were utilized to regulate the levels that were out of balance. (Please note that appropriate guidance should be considered when supplementation is used to remediate neurotransmitter imbalances.) Within a few days on the supplements, Charlie was sleeping better; within the first two weeks, his teachers were noticing a more focused child. By the time he was retested, Charlie had made great strides, and the test results showed that his brain was becoming more balanced.

Every person has a unique neurotransmitter profile. Only the necessary nutrients should be used to balance brain chemistry; general supplementation with all of the amino acids rarely solves imbalances. While single amino acids can work to balance the brain, doing so often requires several different products; such a regimen should also include vitamin and mineral cofactors and a high-quality omega-3 fatty acid. The best supplement protocols incorporate the child's individual requirements and provide a program of highly targeted amino acids specific to the imbalances as verified through lab testing. All of the brain nutrient needs are then combined into a few products, making it easy and convenient to buy and use. Individual protocols can make a measurable difference based on proven testing methods.

Restoring healthy neurotransmitter levels and achieving the correct balance can have a profoundly positive effect on health problems like depression, anxiety, ADD/ADHD, headache, migraines, weak memory, poor focus, chronic pain, and more. However, an expert is required to determine the proper protocol.

Omega-3 fatty acids and multivitamins are also important elements in helping the brain function optimally. Omega-3 fatty acids are vital to restoring brain health by increasing nerve cell signaling, fluidity, and conductivity. They ensure proper communication of nerve cells. Unfortunately, many children and adults don't get sufficient omega-3 fatty acids in their regular diets, so supplementation is commonly used. Recent studies attribute omega-3 fatty acids to improvement in children's mental health. Reduction in autistic and hyperactive behaviors is also common with the use of omega-3 fatty acids, as well as a more balanced mood, decreased anxiety, and a decrease in compulsive behaviors. The B-complex vitamins along with magnesium and certain micronutrients are necessary components for the synthesis of brain chemicals. This is the reason that they are recommended along with amino acid therapy.

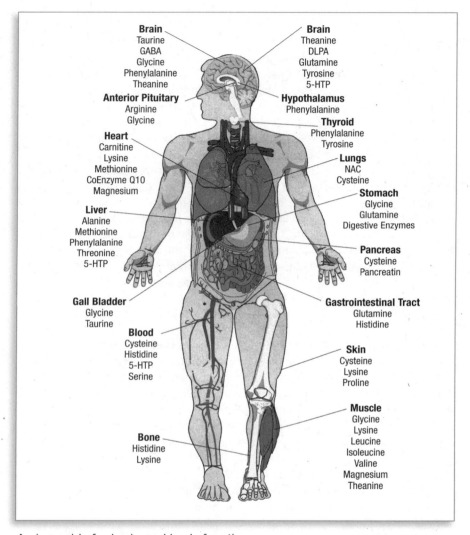

Brain
Taurine
GABA
Glycine
Phenylalanine
Theanine

Anterior Pituitary
Arginine
Glycine

Heart
Carnitine
Lysine
Methionine
CoEnzyme Q10
Magnesium

Liver
Alanine
Methionine
Phenylalanine
Threonine
5-HTP

Gall Bladder
Glycine
Taurine

Blood
Cysteine
Histidine
5-HTP
Serine

Bone
Histidine
Lysine

Brain
Theanine
DLPA
Glutamine
Tyrosine
5-HTP

Hypothalamus
Phenylalanine

Thyroid
Phenylalanine
Tyrosine

Lungs
NAC
Cysteine

Stomach
Glycine
Glutamine
Digestive Enzymes

Pancreas
Cysteine
Pancreatin

Gastrointestinal Tract
Glutamine
Histidine

Skin
Cysteine
Lysine
Proline

Muscle
Glycine
Lysine
Leucine
Isoleucine
Valine
Magnesium
Theanine

Amino acids for brain and body functions.
Reprinted with permission Pain & Stress Publications (San Antonio, TX)

However, many parents are not aware of the benefits omega-3 fatty acids provide. Recent research, conducted by Harris Interactive, reveals that 68 percent of parents in the United States are not sure what omega-3 DHA does, and 59 percent of parents are not aware of the benefits of omega-3 DHA to their child's health. The myelin sheath, or insulation for nerves, is created from omega-3 fatty acids. Children should not be given flaxseed oil, even though it is rich in omega-3 fatty acids, since they do not yet have the correct enzymes to break down the oil to the proper form needed to create the myelin sheath.

Amino Acids and the Adopted Child

Mia is a beautiful seven-year-old who was adopted at the age of two from a rural Russian orphanage. It's presumed that she endured emotional and physical neglect, abuse, and malnourishment. When her parents brought her home, she had burn marks on her back, was severely underweight, and cried constantly; her parents were unable to soothe her despite their best efforts. Even with their unconditional love and regard, Mia would bite, kick, scream, and ignore their attentions. She couldn't tolerate being held or touched by her father. In public she would throw tantrums, and her parents were literally confined to their home.

Professionals eventually diagnosed her with post-traumatic stress disorder (PTSD) and reactive attachment disorder (RAD). These diagnoses are quite common for adoptees. Many of these children receive therapeutic interventions or are prescribed medications to alleviate symptoms. The problem is that with cases such as Mia's, the therapy was only helping her with the presenting behaviors, not the internal causes of these behaviors: her chemical imbalances. She was eventually able to use words when she was upset and talk about her feelings. However, after much time and exhaustion, Mia's meltdowns still occurred daily. She was abusive toward her parents and peers, and was eventually expelled from school. At that point, neurotransmitter testing and amino acid therapy was her parents' last hope before medication.

Attachment is one of the most important aspects of children's development; it is the essential factor in shaping their minds through interactions. Early deprivation, abuse, trauma, and dysfunctional attachment can disrupt children's brain development and, thus, their production and management of neurotransmitters. Research on abused and neglected children indicates the devastating effects of maltreatment on the developing brain: smaller brain size, decreased growth of the corpus callosum (the connective pathway between the right and left sides of the brain), and impaired growth of inhibitory neurotransmitters, including GABA, which serve to calm the excitable emotional limbic structures. This is seen in brain imaging studies and neurotransmitter testing. Even after abused children are introduced into safe and loving homes, the distorted neurochemistry is still present.

Neurotransmitters and Trauma

Inhibitory neurotransmitters develop in infancy and, over time, increasingly develop through touch and having one's needs met; a baby cries to be fed, he's held, and he receives the milk he needs. However, neglect, inappropriate touch, malnourishment, and traumatic events send mixed messages to the brain. Consequently, the brain is unable to develop an optimal amount of these much-needed inhibitory neurotransmitters, which frequently leads to the inability to control responses from excitatory neurotransmitters and contributes to children living in a state of fear and/or hypervigilance.

Excitatory neurotransmitters are dispatched in children who have endured neglect or trauma as a means for them to get their needs met. This is a survival mechanism. They may be the loudest child in the orphanage, use aggression to fight off those who are hurting them, or stay awake in fear of the unknown. Their inhibitory neurotransmitters are not fully developed, so they run on excitatory energy, unable to calm themselves down or develop proper inhibitory support.

When these reserves are exhausted, we start to see the child that Mia has become; although she desperately wants to be loved by her parents, she can't reciprocate that love. Her mind is working in a "fight or flight" modality, she lacks impulse control, and she generally responds out of fear. This isn't Mia's fault or the fault of her parents; it is simply the way her brain developed, making any intervention impossible without balancing the brain first.

Sympathetic and Parasympathetic Nervous Systems

The sympathetic and parasympathetic nervous systems have different but complementary functions. The sympathetic nervous system is responsible for the excitatory messages, and the parasympathetic nervous system is the regulator of the inhibitory neurotransmitters. In other words, the sympathetic division could be considered as the accelerator and the parasympathetic division as the brakes. The sympathetic division typically engages when actions require quick responses. The parasympathetic division engages when actions do not require immediate reactions. When children do not have adequate calming neurotransmitters, they do not have the "brakes" to reduce fear-based, excitatory behaviors.

Putting the Pieces Together

The goal of any therapeutic regimen is to help your child function optimally. Neurotransmitter testing and remediation is one alternative for repairing your child's chemical imbalances naturally. With so many different approaches available today, it can become confusing. To get the most benefit, seek out a program that measures neurotransmitter levels objectively using noninvasive methods. Seek out a practitioner with solid clinical experience who will work with you, review the test results, and provide customized protocols and supplementation. Make sure the plan includes regular follow-up to guide you and your child along the road to brain wellness.

It is important to note that amino acid therapy is effective because testing is available to quantify your child's neurotransmitter levels. Because this is objective testing, it is not a guessing game; the laboratory results speak for themselves. Balancing neurotransmitter levels works in conjunction with other therapies and should be customized for each patient. This may be just one piece in the complicated puzzle of your child's treatment plan, but I believe it is the foundation. Amino acid therapy often enables children to get benefits from other necessary therapies. Regardless of which approach you choose, my hope is that you will heal your child in the most natural and effective manner possible.

—Emily Roberts, MA, LPC-I

ADHD and the Thyroid Gland

If your child is showing symptoms that you think may be attention deficit hyper-activity disorder, don't be so fast to apply that label. There are other conditions that can produce similar symptoms. Before jumping to conclusions, rule out a possible thyroid problem.

While ADHD is the most commonly diagnosed behavioral disorder in children, there are no specific laboratory tests to confirm the diagnosis. The diagnosis is determined by the presence of a variety of symptoms that can include, to varying degrees, inattentiveness, difficulty concentrating, distractibility, hyperactivity, and impulsive behavior. Not everyone with an ADHD diagnosis need display all of these behaviors. Children, especially girls with the inattentive form of ADHD, are often not diagnosed until middle school because of their lack of disruptive behavior. Others may be hyperactive and impulsive but not necessarily inattentive. Recent studies have demonstrated a physiologic basis for this difference.

The thyroid gland produces hormones that are essential for normal brain development. In children, often the earliest indications of an overactive thyroid, called hyperthyroidism, may be behavioral as opposed to physical. Nervousness, a key hyperthyroid symptom, may be expressed in children as hyperactivity. Moodiness, forgetfulness, and inattention are also common symptoms of hyperthyroidism, and all are common features of ADHD as well. Due to a specific gene mutation, some people show a reduced responsiveness to the thyroid hormones, a condition known as generalized resistance to thyroid hormone, or GRTH. Although not a particularly common disorder, about 70 percent of children with this genetic resistance to thyroid hormone exhibit symptoms of ADHD. Furthermore, children with GRTH are more prone to learning disabilities than children with ADHD.

The typical laboratory picture of hyperthyroidism will show high levels of the thyroid hormones triiodothyronine (T3) and thyroxine (T4) and a low level of thyroid stimulating hormone (TSH), which is produced by the pituitary gland and stimulates the thyroid gland when the body senses that more thyroid hormone is needed. In GRTH, levels of T3 and T4 will be high, as in regular hyperthyroidism, but TSH levels will be normal to high.

Researchers studying this phenomenon have shown that the high levels of T3 and T4 are significantly correlated with symptoms of hyperactivity and impulsivity but do not seem to have any correlation to symptoms of inattention or distractibility. Levels of TSH do not correlate significantly with any of the symptoms of ADHD.

When evaluating the thyroid gland to see if it may be involved as a cause of behavioral symptoms similar to ADHD, be suspicious if the lab results don't fit the clinical picture. There have been cases where an unusual antibody that reacts with the standard TSH test gives a false high reading, suggestive of GRTH, when in fact the TSH is actually low.

Given the frustration, not to mention the expense, of evaluating and treating children with ADHD, it makes sense to screen for thyroid problems first, using simple, noninvasive, readily available tests.

—Stuart H. Garber, DC, PhD

Brain Seizures and the ADHD Connection

t's reported that up to 38 percent of kids diagnosed with a seizure disorder have attention disorders. A higher-than-usual incidence of seizures is also seen in those with mental retardation and a variety of other neurobehavioral disorders, such as autism, Tourette's syndrome, and reactive attachment disorder (RAD). Performing an EEG is highly recommended to rule out seizures as a possible cause or contributing factor to ADD/ADHD.

Quantitative electroencephalography (QEEG) is a quantitative computer analysis of brain electrical activity, or brainwaves, which are recorded from sensors placed on the scalp. The EEG procedure has been used in neurology, psychiatry, and other fields of medicine since the 1950s. One of the initial uses of EEG was during sleep, to detect times when a person was motionless and quiet during sleep but had active brain waves (REM sleep). If people were awakened during this time, they often reported they were dreaming. This was one of the first uses of EEG, to peek "below the surface" of behavior and look at the underlying brain processes.

Perhaps the most important feature of EEG is that it measures changes in patterns of brain function and activity over short periods of time, down to milliseconds. In addition, EEG is completely noninvasive and cost effective, and it doesn't involve exposure to radioactive agents, as do SPECT and PET scans.

Medically, EEG recordings are used mostly to determine whether someone has seizures. When most people experience seizures, they do not have grand mal seizures, the kind that cause obvious convulsions, rolling of the eyes, and biting of the tongue. The most common type of seizure is associated with a brief lapse of awareness, known as petit mal seizures or partial seizures. This loss of awareness is often mistaken for inattentiveness in the classroom. The seizure event may not be recognized as a seizure, and instead may be described as "spacing out," "glazing over," or that the person has "spells" of some kind. It's useful to evaluate those experiences with EEG, because seizures are often the culprit.

Causes of seizures are often complex and not well understood. Descriptively, a seizure is a rapid discharge of brain electrical activity. Many seizures do not have any known causes and are therefore referred to as idiopathic. Seizures have a genetic predisposition; that is, they tend to run in families. Other physical causes of seizures include the presence of tumors, cysts, or scarring that causes small regions of the brain to become irritated and produce rapid electrical discharges.

Seizures are usually treated with anticonvulsant medications. The first generation of anticonvulsants included Dilantin, Tegretol, and Depakote. The second generation of anticonvulsants was marketed in the mid-1990s, including Topamax, Gabitril, and Lamictal. Newer anticonvulsants, such as Trileptal, are now appearing on the market. These drugs differ in their mechanisms of action and many are used not only for seizures, but also for psychiatric disorders without evidence of epilepsy. Newer medications tend to yield more specific action and fewer side effects.

New technology known as neurofeedback has been shown to yield positive changes in individuals with epileptic seizures. The early research on neurofeedback was carried out with cats exposed to seizure-producing agents. Rewarding cats to produce certain specific brain rhythms was demonstrated by M. B. Sterman at UCLA to protect the animals from seizures following exposure to these agents. This discovery led numerous researchers and clinicians to explore the use of EEG neurofeedback to treat seizures in humans. Neurofeedback is now used to treat a wide variety of neurobehavioral disorders, and specific procedures for neurofeedback are increasingly guided by the results of QEEG.

The QEEG study involves recording brainwaves using standard clinical procedures. Sensors are placed at specific locations on the scalp and around the eyes. Caps or nets have been outfitted with sensors, so they can be placed quickly and efficiently on the head, rather than one by one at each location. This setup usually takes about fifteen minutes, and the recording takes about another fifteen to twenty minutes. A portion of the recording is made with the person simply resting with his or her eyes closed and eyes opened. Other challenges, such as hyperventilation (heavy breathing) or photic stimulation (flashing lights), are often carried out to provoke abnormalities. Academic or cognitive challenges, such as reading or math problems, are sometimes performed during the recording to look for patterns of task-related activation.

EEG technology has evolved from recording brain waves on paper with ink writers to digitizing the signals and displaying them on a computer screen. Digitizing the EEG is much like everything else that is digitized in our daily lives. We commonly use digital cell phones and digitize pictures and music. Digitizing the EEG is no different. Once the EEG is digitized and stored in the computer, an analysis of the EEG can be performed to generate more information than is available simply by looking at the brain waves.

The QEEG analysis breaks down the complex waveform into frequencies. The results indicate how much of each frequency of the EEG—usually from one to thirty-two cycles per second (Hz)—is present at each sensor. Observations are often made about the correlation between the activity for each sensor and the activity from surrounding sensors. The amount of electrical power and the correlations among sensors are compared to an age-appropriate reference database composed of individuals with no symptoms of neurological or psychiatric disorder to see if there are significant deviations from the "normal" pattern. Where the deviations occur on the head, and how large the deviations are, can also be determined.

A QEEG does not diagnose a behavioral problem, but rather it peeks below the surface to determine what the neurophysiological disturbance underlying the problem might be. When a neurological abnormality is identified, possible intervention strategies can be suggested. Although historically most interventions have used medication, use of neurofeedback and nutriceutical (nutritional) methods to positively influence the activity of the nervous system is increasing. A number of other behavioral training techniques are increasingly being used adjunctively to ameliorate certain behavioral problems, such as the Listening Program for auditory processing, Fast Forward for language encoding, the Interactive Metronome for timing and sequencing, and Heart Rate Variability (HRV) for anxiety.

In summary, the QEEG procedure is an extension of clinical EEG testing and is a complement to tests such as the MRI that image brain structure, not function. The QEEG allows the evaluation of the neurological events underlying behavioral problems. It can help to suggest specific treatment and monitor changes in the nervous system produced by interventions, and is a useful tool in reducing the list of possible root causes for ADD/ADHD.

—*Jack Johnstone, PhD*

Electromagnetic Field Disturbances

As a board-certified family physician and holistic practitioner, I see many patients with ADD and ADHD. To me, this is just a part of the spectrum of autism, with ADD/ADHD situated in the milder array of this complex disorder.

One study that involved over five years of research on children with autism and other membrane-sensitivity disorders found that electromagnetic radiation (EMR) negatively affects cell membranes by causing a change in cell membrane polarity and allows heavy metal toxins, associated with autism, to build up in the body. The charged membrane won't allow the heavy metals in the cells to be drawn out with chelation or detoxification efforts, similar to the way that positive ends of magnets repel each other. The positively charged heavy metals can't escape through the membrane to exit the body. The researchers pointed out that autism rates have increased concurrently with the proliferation of cell phones and wireless use.

Speaking in reference to the huge rise in autism rates, George Carlo, the study's coauthor, said, "A rise of this magnitude must have a major environmental cause. Our data offer a reasonable mechanistic explanation for a connection between autism and wireless technology." The researchers also suggest that EMR from wireless devices works in conjunction with environmental and genetic factors to cause autism.

Most people aren't even aware of electromagnetic field (EMF) problems. When told of some of the symptoms, however, they respond with recognition. Dr. Carlo mentions the following symptoms: inability to concentrate, irritability, insomnia, obsessive ideations, compulsive behavior, anxiety, depression, and headaches, among others. CBS recently reported that cell phone use was being added to the list of items and activities that pregnant women should avoid, along with cigarette smoking and alcohol consumption, due to studies showing a significantly higher incidence of hyperactivity in children born to cell phone users.

A study by Peter Franch found unequivocally that "cells are permanently damaged by cellular phone frequencies." This cellular damage, Franch noted, is maximized at low dosage and "inherited unchanged, from generation to generation." This means that the damaged cells are transmitted for up to four generations by epigenetically modifying gene expression in their offspring.

Dr. Franch also found that the production of histamine, which triggers bronchial spasms, is nearly doubled after exposure to mobile phone transmissions. Cell phones also reduce the effectiveness of antiasthmatic drugs and retard recovery from illness. This means asthma, emphysema, and other lung diseases are worsened significantly by cell phone use.

British military scientists discovered that cell phone transmissions disrupt the brain sites for memory and learning, causing forgetfulness and sudden confusion. Other studies show that electromagnetic signals from cellular phones reduce the ability to concentrate, calculate, and coordinate complicated activities such as driving a car. This is added to the already documented 35 percent involvement of cell phone use in all automobile accidents. Some of the accidents are caused simply by the distractions of listening, dialing, or texting on these devices, and others are caused by the cognitive disruption of the brain from the cell phone itself while the user is driving.

Apart from the microwave oven, mobile telephones are the most radioactive appliance we've ever invented, and people put them right by their heads—arguably the most sensitive part of the body. The pegged needle of a shrieking EMR meter placed beside a connected cell phone still shows significant exposure one hundred feet away. Cell phones emanate microwave radiation, and human brains may absorb up to 60 percent of that energy. Already, there are at least fifteen thousand scientific reports on this subject, some by Russian scientists dating as far back as the 1940s. It has been discovered that small amounts of energy, when delivered in the right way, can have the same effects as a massive dose of chemicals.

The most delicate fields of electromagnetic energy influence the complexity of living creatures. There are sixty-six epidemiological studies showing that electromagnetic radiation across the spectrum increases brain tumors in human populations. Two of those studies are for particular brain tumors from cell phones. Because cancer takes decades to develop, it will be another ten to twenty years before "mobiles" manifest a bonanza in brain tumors. Vini Khurana, a Mayo Clinic-trained neurosurgeon with an advanced neurosurgery fellowship in cerebral vascular and tumor microsurgery from the Barrow Neurological Institute in Phoenix, Arizona, reported in March 2008 that cell phone use is potentially more dangerous than cigarette smoking and that the widespread use of cell phones may be more detrimental to human health than asbestos and cigarettes combined. The types of tumors produced by the low-energy fields are found to be inoperable and very resistant to all known chemotherapies.

Daniel Foggo reported that cancer clusters and other serious illnesses have been discovered around mobile phone masts, raising concerns over the technology's potential impact on health. Studies of the mobile phone mast sites show high incidence of cancer, brain hemorrhages, and high blood pressure within a radius of four hundred yards. This means we are getting damaged by "second-hand cell phone energy," similar to the damage caused by second-hand smoke.

I have clients with breast cancer growing under the area where their cell phones are stored in their purses when the purse is worn, and men with testicular cancer on the side where their phones were pocketed. Thermography (the study of heat distribution) of children's brains while the children are holding a cell phone to their skull shows heat penetrating across to the other side of the brain. These abnormal, low-energy waves create cell damage that results in brain cell apoptosis (premature cell death), especially the stem cells that form replacement cells as a person ages. We will soon have a generation suffering from presenile dementia in epidemic proportions.

I sometimes use a homeopathic remedy from Professional Complementary Health Formulas called Radialgin, or some of the products from BioPro, to normalize EMF damage to the body and allow heavy metals to come out. Metagenics makes a great oral product that increases mercury excretion without all the mineral depletion. It's called MetalloClear and is made from herbs that stimulate the metallothionein enzyme in the mitochondria.

Every disease label (including ADD/ADHD) placed upon children can't do justice to the fact that there is no single cause for these problems. Rather, a wide range of multifaceted components are responsible and need to be individually addressed.

Although this section is primarily concerned with the issue of EMFs, the following briefly covers my thoughts on some of the other contributing factors. Without correcting the majority of relevant issues, no one approach will bring about resolution of the symptoms of ADD/ADHD.

"Life and death begin in the gut" is a naturopathic saying that I was never taught in medical school, but it is as true as anything I ever learned. Stopping food intolerances (if they are present) to dairy products, nightshades, or glutens is one of the first steps. Treating intestinal pathogens, such as *Candida*, parasites, or dysbiosis (an imbalance of "bad" bacteria), and then replacing the bad flora with probiotics ("friendly" bacteria) is the next step.

Vaccines may precipitate certain neuroimmunological catastrophes, but not just because of the thimerosal (a mercury-based preservative). There are up to twenty-three other poisons in vaccine preservatives, such as formaldehyde or acetone, which are known neurotoxins and carcinogens. However, the U.S. Congress has given the pharmaceutical companies a "get out of jail free card," and they are no longer responsible for injuries. Giving multiple vaccines in a short period of time (giving more than one type of vaccination within a three-month period) can evoke a toxic response in children or adults. Only the nasal form of influenza vaccine is free of the thimerosal present in all injectable forms of the flu vaccine. Please read *Vaccines: Are They Safe and Effective?* (New Atlantean Press, 2008) by Neil Anderson, MD, before using vaccines. (The answer to the question posed in the title of his book turns out to be a staggering No!)

Pesticides and other chemicals cause important enzymes in the body to cease functioning; they also induce premature cell death (apoptosis). These pesticides contain large quantities of heavy metals as cofactors in the pesticide's effectiveness. Any heavy metal, but especially mercury, may cause neuropathy and encephalopathy. Search the Web for a video by the University of Calgary on the toxic effects of mercury in dental amalgams, and view it on a day you don't mind having the earth shaken under your feet. Silver amalgams are less than 5 percent silver and more than 70 percent mercury, and they continue to poison the body as long as they are present. Use composite fillings from a dentist certified by the American Academy of Biological Dentistry, not the mercury fillings that are pushed by the American Dental Association.

Next, I look at the way the family metabolizes their essential fatty acids to see if there is any insulin resistance or metabolic syndrome that would indicate the genetic inability to convert alpha-linoleic acid (such as from flaxseeds or fish oil) to good essential fats: eicosapentaenoic acid (EPA) for the cell membranes and docosahexaenoic acid (DHA) for brain/nerve cells. Without DHA, the brain and nerves cannot function. Receptor cells on the brain are made from DHA, and all of my young patients with ADHD, ADD, and autism have this weakness. If the patient is vegan, I prescribe a blue-green algae supplement for their DHA; otherwise I recommend Metagenics EPA-DHA high-concentrate liquid, since it's already broken down for easy assimilation. Cod liver oil and salmon oil are still in the alpha-linoleic acid state, which is not a usable form for them.

I also recognize that many children and adults have detoxification weaknesses. Some respond well to transdermal L-glutathione to help the liver rid the body of toxins. This is especially true in autism, where everyone in this group needs methylated folic acid to enable gamma-aminobutyric acid (GABA) to become dopamine (for focus), L-tryptophan to become serotonin (for mood), and melatonin (for sleep). For this, I personally recommend Metagenics FolaPro twice a day. In most cases, implementing dietary changes along with the use of DHA and FolaPro results in children with ADHD moving from detention hall to the head of the class within three weeks.

ADD/ADHD is on the rise in epidemic proportions. Without adequately addressing exposure to harmful EMFs and other environmental factors, attempts to combat ADD/ADHD stand little chance of success.

—Dan O. Harper, MD

SECTION

V

Alternative Approaches to Healing

ADHD

SPURIOUS DIAGNOSIS, SPECIOUS TREATMENT

n the mid 1960s, I was in graduate school at the University of Wisconsin in Madison. At that time there were only two graduate schools in the country offering programs in what I wanted to study: the effect of neurodevelopmental differences on behavior and learning. Those were exciting days with new concepts mentioned in various research papers: words like "neuroplasticity" and concepts such as "the role of myelination in neuronal processing and brain development." In the Department of Counseling and Behavioral Studies, Division of Behavioral Disorders, specializing in neurological impairments, I was in a position to read the research and engage in projects that tinkered on the edge of breaking discoveries.

It was during that period that a phenomenon was occurring in the United States: the diagnosing of many students with mysterious disorders beyond the more clear-cut syndromes such as autism, Down's syndrome, cerebral palsy, and testable disorders such as dyslexia and dysgraphia. People, especially children, were being diagnosed with attention deficit disorder and also with hyperkinesis (now called hyperactivity). As a hopeful graduate student and an optimistic professional, in the first few years of my career as a learning disabilities specialist, I thought that I would see the development of approaches that would apply those recently discovered phenomena of neurological functioning—discoveries such as the fact that neurons with fatter myelin sheaths processed information more readily and helped the brain integrate sensory input and organize information for a response. Coupled with research from educational psychology showing that repeated organized stimulation helped build strong neural pathways and that overstimulation of immature neural pathways was detrimental, these discoveries promised to yield ways to alleviate many if not most disorders of behavior and learning—not only in children but across the lifespan. I was thrilled to be on the cutting edge, helping to facilitate these improvements.

In my naïve optimism, I did not take into account another factor that was developing even more swiftly—the development of psychotropic medication (mind-altering drugs) to be given not only to adults who were diagnosed with psychiatric disorders, but even to elementary school children who displayed inadequate focus and follow-through on the directions and tasks their teachers or parents gave them. Children who became diagnosed with ADHD were first given Dexedrine with the intent of speeding up their neural processing, so they could take in and process information more rapidly and so they might retain focus. I was appalled. Hadn't the educated populace in the world heard that fatter neural fibers process more readily, and that through the combination of proper nutrition (largely by the inclusion of "good oils"—essential fatty acids) and repeated, organized, nonstressful stimulation, the brain and nervous system adapt themselves and become better equipped to function? Had no one learned the lessons of overstimulation—that it can abuse and shut down the very pathways they are targeting, or that by putting undue stress on immature or irregularly functioning systems (especially the immature visual system), they can cause damage or aggravate adverse responses such as tics? And what about the numerous studies on sleep disturbances and the negative impact they have on all aspects of functioning? Why were the American educational and medical communities pressuring families to put their children at risk by giving them mind-altering drugs?

I went abroad from 1978 to 1989 and was able to study other theories in the fields of education and health care, and to work collaboratively with a wide range of professionals who were employing more holistic approaches to human functioning and less damaging ways of resolving hyperactive behaviors, delayed responses to directions, and difficulties sustaining focused attention. During that period, I developed a comprehensive approach to identify the root causes of many different disorders and to resolve the challenges they presented to individuals of all ages who wanted to function in classrooms and other situations. I named that approach HANDLE, an acronym for Holistic Approach to NeuroDevelopment and Learning Efficiency. But I soon found that, in 1990 in the United States, the public was doubtful that something holistic might be anything other than a spoof, a means to draw desperate families into unresearched therapy that provided only false hope when what they wanted was a real cure. This need for a cure was fed by the fact that parents were led to believe that their five-year-olds' inability to sit still for forty minutes and attend to a lesson or perform operations with a computer program was a sign of a serious disorder. The entire concept of readiness to learn somehow had been forgotten. And educators and parents both seemed to ignore the fact that the visual system is the last system to develop and the slowest to mature, so placing undue demands on the eyes at an early age can be very stressful, especially when the opportunities to rest the eyes by looking into unobstructed expanses become few and far between, with less time outdoors and clutter in the spaces indoors. With the reliance on televisions and computers, another important fact seems to have been ignored: children (and adults) require movement. Equally forgotten or ignored is the fact that movement is synonymous with learning and with life—neural impulse, after all, is movement, as are respiratory and cardiac functions. I was still confused as to how it had happened that the neurological studies of the '60s and even earlier had been buried and that children and adults were being labeled with disorders and then prescribed medication classified as a class II drug, as dangerous as cocaine (which it resembled). Weren't the Federal Drug Administration, the Drug Enforcement Agency, and National Institutes of Health protecting them? In the next couple of years, I was to learn not only why this was occurring but also why the number of children and adults diagnosed with ADD or ADHD was increasing in epidemic proportions, although it was known that there were no viral or other epidemiological reasons for this proliferation.

In 1991, I began to offer presentations and training in communities across the country where anyone would gather a group of open-minded professionals and laypersons interested in hearing about a different model of treating disorders such as ADD, learning disabilities, Tourette's syndrome, autism, and other perplexing concerns. I developed charts and models to explain the functions underlying readiness for and success in learning and other social interactions. In the process, I discussed the importance of nutrition, especially essential fatty acids and water, and explained the effects of toxicity and *Candida albicans* and other concepts the public had not yet become familiar with.

In 1995, not quite a year after I opened The HANDLE Institute in Seattle to provide community information, professional training, and clinical services with a nondrug approach to treat ADD and other neurodevelopmental challenges, the Public Broadcasting System presented the Merrow Report—an exposé on the relationship between Ciba-Geigy (now Novartis) and CHADD (Children and Adults with Attention Deficit Disorders), the largest national nonprofit organization providing support groups and information for parents and teachers of those who were diagnosed with or suspected of having ADD or ADHD. Reports revealed that Ciba-Geigy, the makers of the form of methylphenidate sold under the name Ritalin, had given CHADD in its first two years over a million dollars to provide desperate families with information on the benefits of medication for ADD/ADHD. And they continued to fund the operations of CHADD as it grew in prominence and developed lobbyists to pressure the Drug Enforcement Administration to change the ranking of Ritalin from a hard narcotic to a drug that could be more readily prescribed, even for young children. Ciba-Geigy insisted there was nothing wrong with their supporting this group, as this was a capitalistic country with freedom of speech. Supporting CHADD and controlling their agenda was the best use of the drug manufacturer's marketing money.

In November 1998, I attended and participated in the National Institutes of Health Consensus Conference on Attention Deficit Hyperactivity Disorder in Bethesda, Maryland. The majority opinion at that conference was that ADHD, however one might choose to define it, is best treated by stimulant medication. Recent exposés on the collusion between the drug companies and the "researchers" whose studies are used to support the use of medication in treating such disorders as ADHD now cast distrust on the conclusions purported by the conference and supported by NIH. I was amazed to learn that the majority of the NIH studies on the effects of medication on ADHD had, over the previous decades, been conducted for an average of only three to four months. The only studies available at the end of 1998 that were called "long term" had occurred in 1997 and had extended for a mere eighteen months.

In response to those of us at the conference who opposed the reliance on medication, some of the specialists chosen to form the consensus report acknowledged that they did not see value in education and rehabilitation services in the treatment of ADHD, and therefore insurance coverage of such services is not necessary. I calmly told them in the public forum that I hoped they would soon realize that those very services are the avenues by which we can effect a real and lasting difference.

The panel agreed that there were no valid diagnostic tests for the assessment of ADHD and yet felt that the diagnoses being made were reliable. This statement confused the scientist in me. I did not know how to respond to such an obvious inconsistency being presented in defense of what is touted as scientific exploration. There were frequent references to the "comorbidity"—that is, presence of other disorders as well—found in children with ADHD. This was the first statement that prompted me to grab a microphone and address the conference.

I received applause for the two-pronged question I posed to the group: First, in light of the comorbidity of ADHD, learning disabilities, obsessive-compulsive disorder, oppositional defiant disorder, anxiety, and depression, does this not imply that there are clusters of symptoms that stem from various weaknesses or immaturities in neurophysiological subsystems and their interaction with other subsystems, and in the discrepancy between the individual's behaviors and subjective expectations on specific tasks in specific situations? And, second, does this not mandate us to seek not only ways to diagnose but also methods to resolve the root causes—in the individual and in the environment—rather than seeking more ways to merely mask the symptoms and control behaviors?

On the last morning of the conference, the consensus statement (see http://odp.od.nih.gov/consensus/cons/110/) revealed that, after many years of expensive studies, NIH is still unable to discern what ADHD is, how to diagnose it, and how to treat it. I once again was given the microphone. I asked those convened if they can entertain the idea that there is no such thing as an attention deficit disorder, since everyone is always attending to something. Differences in our neurophysiological makeup, our emotional status, and other factors make it more or less difficult for us to set and sustain our attention on what someone else considers the task at hand. I then invited them to join HANDLE in renaming the issue we were examining and call it attentional priority disorder (APD). With this major change in perspective, the true problem can come into focus and be dealt with systemically, holistically, fully.

One of the concluding statements in the consensus report was that a major problem in finding appropriate treatment and services for ADHD was lack of information, particularly regarding alternative approaches. I wished to address this point as well but did not have the chance. My statement would simply have been that there is no lack of information; but there *is* a lack of information readily available to the public because political and commercial funding supports a specific agenda only.

Now, in 2008, we are at a crossroads. We have two elements to thank for this. First, the other "epidemic" that has taken hold of society and is now discussed and studied more than ADHD: autism and the autism spectrum disorders. Autism was enough of a challenge to the educational and medical communities in 1965 for the Autism Society of America to emerge in an attempt to solve the puzzle of this confusing syndrome. By 1995, diagnoses of autism were escalating across the country and around the world. The focus to find the cause and the cure for autism has led to a profound change of attitude in the minds of those touched by and studying this new epidemic. The realization that there is no one explanation—not genetics, not nutrition, not allergies, not numerous other factors studied—has led to the need to explore a total load theory. Holism, at last, is finding a place in scientific and medical exploration!

And another remarkable thing has happened. The media has suddenly taken an interest in what they are touting as new concepts: neuroplasticity (with its numerous implications) and the role of the environment in the formation of neural pathways. With the realization that the human being and its many systems are in a constant state of interaction with the environment and that each person's systems are influenced by the numerous elements in his or her life situation (including, of course, genetic predispositions to certain factors), perhaps there is now the readiness to look deeper into my concept of attentional priority disorders. Granted, there is no formal scientific research to support most of the work I and other HANDLE providers have done in exploring this area and in helping thousands of families around the world to understand it and to resolve the challenges. However, the validity of much of the published research has become questionable with the recently and blatantly exposed collusion between drug companies and medical researchers of high esteem—researchers whose actions have cast aspersion on the studies and ethics of such eminent institutions as the Harvard Medical School. It is time to review the HANDLE paradigm and judge its applicability to ADHD and other disorders as well.

A Holistic Understanding

Up until this point, I have been discussing labels: ADD, ADHD, autism, and even attentional priority disorder. However, no one can treat labels. What we can treat are the root causes of the symptoms that cluster together into the basis for a diagnosis or label. To truly understand the root causes of dysfunctional behaviors, we must look beyond the label at the behaviors themselves. Behaviors are communication, telling us what systems are irregular or immature or distressed, when we know how to discern the sensory-motor systems that the behaviors express. By combining observational assessment with in-depth information from a developmental profile, we can determine connections among each individual's systems and develop appropriate nondrug interventions that truly change the structure and function of the brain.

Not only are labels like ADD and ADHD limiting, they may not accurately reflect the experiences of a child (or adult) diagnosed with these conditions. By changing the focus to APD, we recognize that no one has a deficit of attention. We are all always attending to something, even in our sleep. The question then becomes what stimuli the person is driven to focus on frequently, to the exclusion of others and to the detriment of his or her ability to sustain focus on the task at hand. The ability to organize sights, sounds, tactile sensations, movement, proprioception, odors, and other stimuli taken in by the senses is somehow compromised in children diagnosed with ADD/ADHD. Their subsequent struggle to feel at ease in their surroundings, in their clothing, and even in their own skin absorbs their attention and takes priority over the acknowledged expectation that they stay in their seats, heed directions, remain focused on schoolwork, or otherwise comply with someone else's priorities. Frequently, information on irregularities during sleep yields the most accurate information on what is distracting or annoying (e.g., inability to tolerate a top sheet on the bed, need for music or a fan in the background), since many children learn early to block annoying sensations so they *can* focus their attention. Yet some of their energy and attention is therefore spent on the act of not feeling the offending clothing or not hearing the irritating sound, and they also may not take in other important information from their tactile or auditory senses, or they may be so stressed that they cannot sustain the activity of paying attention for a prolonged period.

Another avenue to gain clues regarding weaknesses in bodily systems is through the ancient technique of reflexology—a method documented in Egyptian and Chinese for more than four thousand years. This system relies on meridians of energy that connect our body from our head to our toes and go into every organ. The feet, hands, and outer ears are the three main surfaces on which we can access these energy channels. By studying the tendencies in the use of our hands and feet, we can gain many helpful clues, but only if we are willing to employ a holistic systems approach to human functionality. For example, a child who holds a pencil in a tripod grasp, with the tip of his thumb on the pencil, but whose thumb immediately flicks up to avoid touching the pencil once it contacts the writing surface because it provides annoying feedback to the sensitive finger tip—that child (like the child who cannot tolerate the top sheet on a bed) is signaling that tactile input is annoying and distracting and that some of his energy is diverted to protect himself from this vulnerability. We all, consciously or not, try to set up situations to protect ourselves in areas of vulnerability.

Individuals with attentional priority disorders may be highly sensitive to sights, sounds, tactile sensations, or odors in their environment, and the expanse of that surround may extend beyond that which is normally perceived. Someone moving a piece of paper many feet from a child who is hypersensitive to touch may truly be disturbing the tactile sense of her classmate. The classmate may not be able to attend to directions or to focus his eyes on his work because he needs to sustain vigilance, a protective readiness in a fright-fight-flight or freeze reaction to this distant and innocent threat of assault. Once anyone has engaged this response, his or her autonomic nervous system takes control, since survival is more important than achievement, and reason temporarily is not an available function. When this occurs, our brain and body work together to take our basic building blocks—

amino acids and other nutrients—and use them to support the stress response, since survival is more important than understanding a lesson in mathematics. Sensory overload in this and other ways can cause the individual to shut down and turn off her attention. If "attack" on the child's irregular senses continues, she may move beyond shutdown to what has been termed a meltdown.

Again, the HANDLE perspective prefers a different term—one that encourages us to look beyond the behavior to the root cause. By calling this behavior a flare-up instead of a meltdown, we will respond as we might to a motorist putting a flare on the side of the road, signaling the need for help in resolving a problem. If we simply suppress the behaviors without learning what is behind them (e.g., employ medication or behavior modification), we may never learn the root cause of the distress, which will fester and reveal itself later, again and again, in other ways.

One of the more common and frequently overlooked reasons for flare-ups relates not to our senses, which bring us information from the external environment, but to nutritional deficits and irregularities that are felt from within. Of course, when both bombardment by external stimuli and nutritional deficits occur simultaneously, the reactions are bound to be more extreme. Some of these nutritional deficits from hypoglycemia (spikes and dips in blood sugar caused by diets high in carbohydrates and low in protein) to more global malnutrition caused by leaky gut syndrome (frequently a result of previous overreliance on antibiotics that have created an overgrowth of *Candida albicans* in the intestinal tract) are discussed in depth in other chapters and must be considered in any holistic approach. The relationship between intestinal health and neural processing is attributable, to a large degree, to the fact that the very neurotransmitters we need for efficient functioning (including input, processing, memory, organization, and response) are made of amino acids—protein—and the protein ingested is not available for use when a leaky gut has allowed it to pass into the bloodstream without proper processing.

Interestingly, the main reason many children have been given repeated antibiotics is for the treatment of ear infections. It is the ear that in so many ways is central to the behaviors that are required for sustained attention and that are irregular in most people with attentional disorders. Of course, the ear helps us hear, and hopefully we can focus that hearing on the directions and discussions to which others want us to attend. The inner ear, comprised of the cochlea (which helps us hear), three bony semicircular canals, and three soft tissue sacs that together comprise the vestibular system and help us orient our bodies in space and control the speed of our movements, also has the awesome job of regulating virtually everything we do! It is responsible for providing the energy for all of our senses other than our three most primal senses of smell, taste, and touch. However, it also interrelates with these senses, because it allows us to respond to them by moving toward or away from pleasant or aversive stimuli, respectively.

Many individuals with attentional disorders have a poor sense of equilibrium and actual physical challenges in supporting or controlling their movements. They may respond impulsively, without accurate or appropriate modulation, or may need to rock, spin, tip back in their chair, or push off from surfaces to provide their brain what it needs to feel secure. Those movements help them pull together the input from many senses, input we are asked to process and form into a coherent perception.

The various sensory and motor systems that are part of our central nervous system include (but are not limited to) olfaction (smelling), gustation (tasting), tactility (touching), vision (seeing), audition (hearing), muscle tone (each muscle's readiness to respond to stimuli), kinesthesia (the sense of movement), and proprioception (the sense of body in space). Each of our primary senses relies on input from different forms of energy (odor/smell, taste, touch, light, sound, pressure, movement), and the brain's job is to differentiate which of the myriad of stimuli impinging on the body and resonating inside the body's internal organs are essential to heed in order to perform the task at hand. If one of those internal organs signals hunger, the need to urinate, or difficulty breathing, those are given priority. When the internal organs become stressed, our body frequently signals us in obvious ways. When one of our processing modalities of differentiation (sorting out relevant from irrelevant input and output), lateralization (the organizing factor of having a dominant eye, hand, leg, ear), and interhemispheric integration (the coordination of both movement and thought patterns of both sides of the body and the brain) is weak, we frequently push ourselves to try a little harder, and we do this until we actually stress some of our internal organs—frequently our respiratory system, resulting in breathing challenges that then interfere with the oxygenation we need for focus, sustained activity, and clear thinking. These interrelationships among our various systems are inextricable and demand a holistic approach.

When these systems truly function well together, the person can function "normally." The diagnosis of ADD/ADHD, Asperger's syndrome, Tourette's syndrome, dyslexia, autism, and other neurological disorders may occur depending on (1) which of these systems is compromised or not connecting efficiently to other systems, (2) the severity or the weakness within any given neurological system(s) or interaction among systems, and (3) the age of onset of the irregularity.

The neural pathways of the central nervous system, including the brain and other organs and systems, use a variety of processing modes to transmit information gathered through our sensory systems, including those in our viscera. They interface our past (memory), present (sensory-motor), and future (intention and aspiration) to give us appropriate plans for action, such as reading, speech, reasoning, writing, movement or refraining from movement, or other responses. When the neural pathways are not well developed and are insufficiently myelinated, messages tend to be transported at a sluggish rate, causing "traffic jams" and sensory overload. If new messages are en route while previous messages have not yet been processed, confusion results. The brain and the rest of the central nervous system become overwhelmed and shut down, just as any thoroughfare when traffic is heavier than the roads can accommodate. When a person is operating in a confused and overwhelmed state, and continued demands are made on his systems, emotional flare-ups occur. The child responds with frustration and anger at his inability to concentrate, to comprehend, to meet the demands of the situation, and to be proud of himself and make others proud of him and his accomplishments.

This is frequently the result of a compromised vestibular system (inner ear) that is unable to simultaneously support vision, hearing, movement, and proprioceptive awareness, all of which are necessary in order first to feel safe and secure and then to respond appropriately to a task in a reasonable amount of time. Additionally, overstimulation of a hypersensitive and/or disorganized system may feel like an assault, in which case the child may respond reactively or even reflexively, rather than responsively.

Outward Behaviors Reflect Inner Challenges

Observing a person's behaviors can offer insight into his or her neurological challenges, if you know what to look for and how to interpret what you see. And there are many signs we can use. For example, if a person looks away from you when you talk to her, she may be signaling you that the challenge of sustaining eye contact detracts from her ability to listen. If she turns away or closes her eyes when she is trying to recall something, she may be telling you that she cannot focus on the pictures in her head against the backdrop of visual input from her physical surrounding. Imploring this child to sustain eye contact can interfere with her ability to attend to the external world, her internal perceptions, or both. No wonder she gets frustrated when she is trying to focus and attend and recall and perform, and is continually distracted by conflicting demands by those very people who want her to focus and attend and recall and perform.

The child who wears a visor or places his hand over his brows may be telling you that his eyes are sensitive to light; fluorescent lights, the reflective lights from screens, and the contrast of black print on shiny white paper distress his visual system. The child drumming with his pencil or fingers on the desktop or constantly moving and fidgeting may be telling us that his inner ear isn't working properly and, in order to pay attention, he must move to keep his vestibular system engaged—not unlike the person who needs to chew gum to stay focused or calm.

Aha! The role of chewing again comes to the fore—not just for its role in digestion, as mentioned earlier, but also for its role in attention. As anyone who has worn braces or experienced other serious dental work will attest, when our teeth are bothering us, it is almost impossible to concentrate on anything else. Why should one little irritated tooth have that much power over our concentration? The answer lies in the largest of our twelve cranial nerves—the trigeminal nerve (the nerve involved in root canal work). It goes into each of our teeth as well as the tongue, cheeks, lips, middle ear, eyebrows, forehead, scalp, nose, and even the cornea of our eyes. It is the culprit for those people who sense they are allergic to the sun, since they sneeze (three times) when they first go out to bright sunlight. What happens is the trigeminal nerve picks up on the heat and light of the sun, and in a fleeting moment of disorganization and being overwhelmed, it sends the message through other segments and branches of the nerve to the nose and the mouth, and the response is sneezing. By the time the person has sneezed for the third time, the system has realized its error and the message gets channeled correctly to the brain to say "ah, sunlight."

With this minimal understanding of the trigeminal nerve (one of the many aspects of our interdependent and interactive systems that is worthy of much more discussion than this space allows), it might become evident why most first- and second-grade students who are losing their baby teeth and getting their permanent teeth have difficulty sustaining their attention on class work, and why teens whose braces have just been adjusted have difficulty studying for their math test. It may also provide us insight into why people who need orthodontia are having trouble accepting the attentional priorities of others. Whether it is in reference to the trigeminal nerve or other tactile sensitivity—or proprioceptive, auditory, vestibular, nutritional, or any other irregularity—the basic rule we need to internalize is that until a child (or an adult) can attend to the neurological challenges dictated by his unique set of circumstances, he won't be able to pay attention to what others define as the task at hand.

Safety and survival are by necessity our highest priorities. Individuals with attentional priority disorders have varying areas of vulnerability, which often surface via strange and disruptive behaviors—an unconscious attempt to sift through and organize the onslaught of information that seems to be bombarding them from all sides. Through HANDLE programs, neurologically challenged children and adults alike can become capable of prioritizing their attention and controlling their behavior, and do this without drugs, once the health of the vestibular system and other neural pathways and systems is established.

Distinguishing Features of HANDLE

Like other natural and alternative health solutions, HANDLE addresses the cause of a problem rather than merely treating symptoms. In other chapters of this book, there is a wealth of information on varied possible reasons that neurological systems can be compromised and on other nondrug approaches that are available to support true healing. While some of these other approaches address issues like toxicity levels and nutritional deficiencies of the brain from a biological perspective, HANDLE uses observational assessment to analyze deficiencies in neurological function by tracing behaviors back to their root causes.

The organized movements in the activities that HANDLE offers engage these neural pathways as harmonious systems, thereby strengthening them, naturally. An activity might involve hopping on one leg and then the other in a certain pattern, thus engaging the vestibular system and cerebellum, which affect balance, muscle tone, and differentiation of one muscle group from another (a necessary part of reflex integration); use of the brain's left and right cerebral hemispheres; and other senses and systems as well, depending on the total environment in which the activity is performed. Continually altering the activities slightly as the individual's systems adapt and improve allows the certified HANDLE practitioner to guide targeted improvements in compromised neurological pathways and systems so, through neuroplasticity, the nervous systems (including the brain) enhance and repair themselves—and ultimately improve the behaviors that are supported by these neurological functions.

One retroactive outcome study available at www.handle.org demonstrated a 90 percent success rate for those families who followed their individualized home-implemented programs, requiring approximately thirty minutes daily. The key factors that underpin HANDLE and lead to its success include the following:

1. A comprehensive holographic understanding of how the numerous neurological systems and the brain function—independently and together, including the hierarchy of interaction among those systems.

2. An artful combination of numerous disciplines, melding Western neuroscientific research with some Eastern healing principles, while maintaining a nonjudgmental, client-centered approach in which behaviors are viewed as communication.

3. An ability to observe an individual and, through the observation of performance and numerous tasks presented, come to a quite accurate conclusion as to which neurological systems/interactions are compromised.

4. A deep understanding that weakened neurological systems can be stimulated only so much before they will become overwhelmed and shut down. This principle of not stressing the systems is referred to as Gentle Enhancement® and is central to all HANDLE programs.

5. A neurodevelopmental/educational approach that provides the client family with an effective, individualized, nondrug program consisting of HANDLE's therapeutic activities, employing Gentle Enhancement, through which neurologic functioning is strengthened without producing stress. These activities are supplemented by complementary suggestions of ways to improve nutritional status, decrease toxic load, and generally strengthen the cellular basis of the client's neurophysiological status.

Earlier in this section, you learned that the collection of symptoms that lead to a diagnosis of ADD/ADHD would be better categorized as attentional priority disorder since the individual's attention is called away from what others define as the task at hand. Similarly, other labels, such as autism, Asperger's syndrome, Tourette's syndrome, bipolar disorder, sensory processing disorder, and dyslexia are also characterized by compromised neurological systems that have multiple causes and are different from person to person. The HANDLE approach recognizes that each individual labeled with a medical diagnosis has a unique set of neurological challenges that can be discerned through observational assessment and intensive interviews. The goal of such assessments according to the HANDLE paradigm is to determine which neurological systems are compromised, and then to provide an individualized treatment plan designed to organize the affected areas and create function from dysfunction.

The recommended activities are simple to perform and require virtually no special equipment. Each person's program is specially designed to meet his or her unique needs, as outlined on the neurodevelopmental profile created by the practitioner with information obtained in the assessment. There are scores of activities, each designed to rely on certain functions while developing others. Some of the most frequently recommended activities involve deceptively simplistic movements, such as the following:

- performing intense sucking with eyes open or closed, depending on what particular challenges a person's visual system may be experiencing
- rhythmic ball bouncing in specific patterns
- systematic tapping on the pathways of the trigeminal nerve
- moving through mazes of varying construction

For individuals with compromised neurological systems, the proper application of these and other activities will steadily improve the functionality of irregular systems. Thousands of satisfied HANDLE clients around the world attest to that, achieving significant gains usually within three to six months, and sometimes as rapidly as a few weeks. Trying to attain a quick fix, however, is one of the reasons that so many people have been lured to find a magic bullet, which has led to an imprudent reliance on medication, causing sudden surges of stimulation that are now being shown to have serious side effects with long-term use. It is possible that through misguided educational and medical speculations that there are critical periods in development, parents have been lured to seek immediate and rapid improvements in functions so that children will not lose out on the supposedly short window of time in which they can develop and learn.

One of the cornerstones of HANDLE, based on long-standing research in neurology and development, is that given the appropriate stimulus and strength of stimulation, neural pathways and neurological systems—including the brain—will adapt, grow, repattern, and repair. HANDLE philosophy places emphasis on proper vestibular functioning (and for that, on adequate lymphatic flow throughout the body) because it is foundational to the functioning of many other neurological systems.

It is not coincidental that a vast majority of children labeled with ADD/ADHD also had recurrent ear infections, given that ear infections, at least temporarily, compromise the vestibular system, and when this happens in formative years, other systems do not receive the integration needed to support optimal development. This leads us to one of the most important clues in rehabilitation: there are *optimal* periods in which development will support ease in social, academic, and motor learning, but it is a mistake to think that these are *critical* periods. Neuroplasticity and common sense support the fact that we continue to develop throughout our lifespan.

What this translates to for each person and family and for humankind is that change, and therefore hope, is eternal. Naturally! And while there is no immediate financial benefit for any corporation or individual that supports natural approaches to healthy neurological functioning and learning, the long-term gains for each family and for our society as a whole are immense. We can be empowered and get a HANDLE on ADD/ADHD, autism spectrum disorders, and so many other maladaptive conditions.

—Judith Bluestone

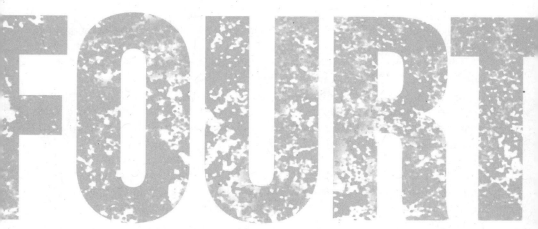

A CHIROPRACTIC NEUROLOGIST'S APPROACH

When Manny first came into the office, his parents and his teacher were at their wits' end. His teacher was upset because Manny tended to fidget in his seat and lose track of what was going on. He always seemed to be fooling around and talking to his friends. He would blurt out answers when he was supposed to be quiet and usually turned in his homework late and half done, if at all. He tended to play the clown and seemed to enjoy disrupting her class. She had told his parents that they needed to put him on drugs for ADHD. His parents were upset because they knew something was wrong but did not want to give Adderall to their twelve-year-old son. They knew he could be a pain, but they also knew that he was a very bright, if unfocused, kid and hoped that there was another way that did not involve drugs.

Sarah is a very pleasant, quiet girl who generally got passing grades. Her teacher appreciated that she never caused trouble, even though she often seemed to be off in a world of her own. She did worry a little about Sarah's poor handwriting and her difficulties in the reading circle, but as long as Sarah was well behaved, she had other problems to deal with. Sarah's few friends and the other kids thought she was sweet but kind of spacey and aloof. Her parents were concerned because she often got headaches, earaches, and tummy aches. They were also concerned because Sarah's language and social development seemed to be a little behind the curve, and she often preferred to play by herself rather than playing with the other kids.

David had already been thrown out of two schools and was on the verge of being expelled from the third. He seemed to enjoy getting into fights and trouble, and while he clearly knew right from wrong, he simply did not seem to care. His father wasn't sure what to do with him—he was too young to be sent to the marines but old enough that the trouble he was flirting with was starting to become serious. If he wasn't such a charmer, he probably wouldn't have gotten away with half the stunts he had already pulled, and his father was worried that he was going to end up seriously injured, arrested, or worse.

These three kids are representative of three different types of attention deficits that each involve different parts of the brain. All of the ADD/ADHD types involve dysfunction in the area of the brain called the prefrontal cortex, and they may involve other areas of the brain as well. There are at least three different parts of the prefrontal cortex that can be dysfunctional. Which ones are involved makes all the difference in the types of symptoms that people experience.

They are named according to the part of the prefrontal cortex involved: ventromedial, dorsolateral, and orbitofrontal. "Ventro" means in front and "dorso" means in back. "Medial" means to the center (of the brain) and "lateral" means out toward the side. "Orbito" means behind the eye and, in this context, "frontal" refers to the frontal lobe of the brain.

Ventromedial Attention Deficits

Sarah is a good example of the ventromedial type of ADD. Ventromedial problems show up as disorders of drive and motivation. Their hallmarks are inattention, apathy, lack of ambition, lack of interest in social interaction, and lack of spontaneity in speech.

People with ventromedial ADD tend to have focus and attention problems, forget what they were doing, and forget to do important things like pay the utility bills, which can drive their family nuts. They tend to have reading problems, easily losing their place, and are often diagnosed with dyslexia.

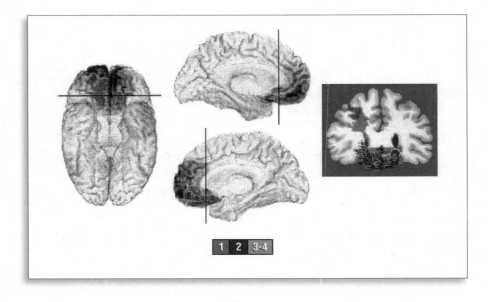

They will often have deficits in social knowledge, especially difficulty interpreting nonverbal emotional expressions. This has also been recognized as contributing to the aberrant social behavior observed following ventromedial prefrontal cortex injuries. This combination makes it challenging for them to develop friends and may be at the root of their preferring their own company.

Dorsolateral ADHD

Manny is a classic example of the dorsolateral type of ADHD. The dorsolateral area of the prefrontal cortex supports executive functions. Problems here usually show up as difficulties with "executive" or goal-directed behaviors. When we think of classic ADHD kids, these are the people we most often think of.

They exhibit poor organizational strategies and frequently have problems with the following tasks:

- planning and sequencing
- thinking ahead
- following complex directions
- anticipating outcomes and consequences
- picking up social cues
- coordination
- rhythm and timing

You can recognize dorsolateral ADHD people by their behaviors:

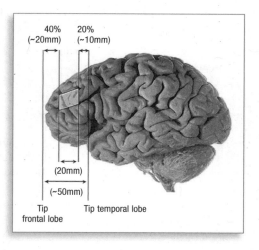

- They start a lot of projects but never seem to get around to finishing them.
- These are often people who don't think about the consequences of their actions until it's too late. They are not bad guys; they just tend to get in trouble because their lack of planning and sequencing results in "ready-fire-aim" kinds of problems. (Wiley Coyote is their poster boy.)
- Although their behavior is often infuriating to those around them, they can often get away with it because they tend to be charming, humorous, and good at manipulating others.
- They will engage in risky behaviors (sex, sports, gambling, business) because the stimulation makes their brain feel good. Consequently, they can end up with drug and alcohol problems.
- They may end up in trouble with their families, their work, or the law because they keep seeking edgier and edgier thrills to excite or stimulate their brains.

Orbitofrontal Attention Deficits

David is typical of someone with orbitofrontal ADHD. Orbitofrontal problems are the most worrisome for society because they create sociopaths. These are the people who know right from wrong, and they know that there are consequences to their actions, but they just don't care. They tend to be unusually distractible and unable to inhibit or filter outside stimuli. They also tend toward inappropriate or childish humor. Their lack of inhibition of instinctual behaviors can lead to belligerence, hypersexuality, and hyperphagia.

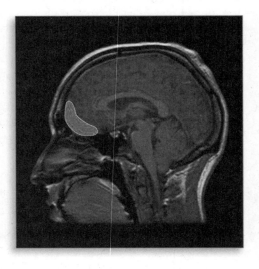

Our jails are filled with people with orbitofrontal problems because they lack conscience. Most of the criminals who have been tested have been found to fit into this group.

The "Where" and the "What" Parts and Vigilance

Another way of looking at what is going on in ADHD is to consider the "where" and the "what" parts of the brain and vigilance. The posterior (back of the brain) attention system is the oldest and most primitive of the three. This is the "where" system that processes stimuli from a particular location so that our attention is reflexively drawn to that location to find out where the stimulus is coming from. Think of our response to the crackle of dry sticks in the woods at night or the attraction of a bright, shiny object in our peripheral vision. This is a very reactive and defensive type of attention.

The anterior (front of the brain) develops the "what" system. This allows us to use memory and factual knowledge based on our internal and external cues to control and focus our attention. It allows us to discriminate the mew and purr of a kitten from the roar of a lion and choose a reasonable and measured response. As our brain grows and develops properly, the newer "what" system should inhibit the primitive "where" system and help us focus our attention by quieting the effects and distraction of external stimuli.

Vigilance is our response to an anticipated threat. This directly inhibits (shuts down) the prefrontal cortex and the "what" system. When we are fearful or vigilant, our vision and hearing are immediately drawn to anything that comes into our environment as we try to discern whether it is a threat or danger to us. We lose the ability to focus, and our reactions default to the "where" system. When you are stuck in the "where" part of the program, busy trying to avoid injury and ostracism, when you are trying to find adequate food and shelter and trying to acquire the Maslow basics, it is difficult to focus on creating the "safe space" to learn new skills that are not involved in immediate survival.

So, how do we calm down the "where" so that the "what" can take over? By turning on the parts of the brain that are snoozing when they should be awake and balancing the parts that are already working.

From the perspective of chiropractic neurology, there are a lot of ways of doing this. Our brain has some wonderful "sensory" systems that are designed to recognize and respond to the world around us. By using tools like sound, light, touch, and smell that turn these sensory systems on, we can bring balance and function into the prefrontal cortex and elsewhere in the brain without using drugs. Two of the most remarkable technologies available to us include Interactive Metronome (IM) training and Retained Primitive Reflex therapy (RPR).

IM training works directly with the brain to turn on the parts that are dormant so that they can create balance and reduce the symptoms of each of the three prefrontal cortex problems described above. We began using Interactive Metronome training in our office in 2001 and have seen remarkable clinical improvements in a broad range of people with autistic spectrum and attention deficit disorders. It is so powerful that we have used IM to turn brain areas back on after traumatic brain injuries and strokes. By improving physical and mental coordination, planning and sequencing, and timing and rhythm, IM is able to vastly improve focus, attention span, and distractibility. We typically see students increase their math and reading comprehension, brain processing, and decision-making speed on standardized tests like the Woodcock-Johnson test by several grade levels (school years) over a matter of several weeks. It is very gratifying to see kids start to focus, interact socially, perform better in school and sports, and start making wiser decisions for themselves.

Angela was one of the more dramatic cases that IM helped. She was fifteen and had already dropped out of school and had had a miscarriage when her mother brought her in for IM. Clearly she was well on her way to not-good things. After five weeks of IM training over the summer, she went back to school in September, where she started making a new and healthier group of friends. She also started using her head in the classroom. Instead of her old D-plus average, she was getting As and Bs when we last heard from her. IM did not give Angela the self-respect or the study skills that turned her world around. It simply turned on parts of her brain so that she could do it from within.

IM looks deceptively simple. Trainees wear a set of stereo headphones and a hand or foot trigger attached to a computer. The computer generates a steady beat fifty-four times per minute, and the trainee attempts to tap their hand or foot right on the beat. The computer measures to within 1/1,000 of a second how far ahead or behind the beat they responded and quickly generates a second tone that tells them how far off the beat they were. If they were ahead of the beat they hear the sound in the left ear, if behind the beat they hear it in their right ear. This gives them the information to adjust their efforts on the next beat. Over the course of several sessions, their brains get turned on and learn, much like the process our brain once went through when we were learning the balance it takes to ride a bicycle.

Through the process of stimulus → response → feedback → correction, the parts of the brain that we are concerned with are turned on and tuned in with the rest of the brain. Specific exercises can aim the IM training at specific brain areas, so the training is individually designed for each trainee.

Retained Primitive Reflex therapy helps move the brain from instinctual "where" reactiveness and vigilance to the "what" state of learning and choosing our response to the world around us. When we are born, our cortex, or main brain, is not fully functional yet, so we rely on our brainstem, or "primitive brain," for our survival. This is where our instinctual or primitive reflexes come in. They happen automatically, instinctually, and outside of our control as survival responses to stimuli from the environment. Since the greatest and most consistent environmental stimulus we face from cradle to grave is gravity, it is not surprising that these are also connected to our relationship with gravity. These reflexes should disappear (integrate) into the developing nervous system during the first year of life, making way for postural reflexes and cognitive functions as the main brain develops. If a primitive reflex remains after its normal age of integration, it becomes a *retained* primitive reflex and can then interfere with the development of balance, postural reflexes, and intentional processes like learning, social skills, and attention.

In natural medicine, we think in terms of the "pyramid of health," which has three sides and a base. The base is structure, and the three sides are biochemistry, neurology, and mental/emotional/spiritual. Retained primitive reflexes, or RPRs, can interfere with all four of these aspects of our life and health. We find them in *all* of the autistic, ADHD, and learning-disabled kids we work with at the Brain Performance Center. They can also reemerge, or be "regained," following neurological, biochemical, emotional, or physical trauma. We especially see this with adult post-traumatic stress disorder, environmental illness, post-stroke, and traumatic brain injury patients. The RPRs seem to most affect the "where versus what" system by locking us into instinctual reactions to stimuli, similar to the hide, fight, or flight responses that we might go to if we heard a sudden noise in the woods at night.

The first RPR is called the fear paralysis reflex (FPR), and it instinctively makes us freeze and be silent, similar to what a rabbit or deer does when startled. This is an ancient reaction that once probably kept us from getting eaten by bigger animals, since most sight-hunters (lions, wolves, bears) work from motion. This same instinctive message to Freeze! can show up as anxiety and panic attacks and social fears and phobias of all types in modern people.

The second RPR is called the moro reflex, and this is the other side of the coin from FPR. Where fear paralysis makes us to try to hide, moro reflex is the "fight or flight" reflex. This is the "where" response in all its glory, blocking the "what" response while dealing in the moment with "survival issues." Retained moro reflexes are usually seen in people with ADHD (especially the classic dorsolateral type), aggressive (type A) personalities, asthma, and a range of sympathetic nervous system dominant problems like adrenal fatigue and digestive, sleep, immune, and hormonal problems.

The following table will give you an idea of some of the problems we see with the different RPRs.

PRIMITIVE REFLEX	SOME PROBLEMS RELATED TO RETENTION
Fear Paralysis Reflex (anxiety, panic attacks, SIDS)	parasympathetic ANS issues
Moro Reflex (Aggression, ADHD, Asthma)	sympathetic ANS issues
Palmar Reflex	verbal and written expression, fine motor skills, posture
Asymmetric Tonic Neck Reflex	learning difficulties, misjudge distances, shoulder injuries
Tonic Labrynthine Reflexes	motion sickness, learning disabilities, balance and visual disturbances
Spinal Galant Reflex	hyperactivity, bedwetting, scoliosis, gait abnormalities
Rooting Reflex	hormonal functions in the HPA axis, including thyroid
Juvenile Suck Reflex	chewing, swallowing, speech, and articulation problems

Fortunately, "fixing" RPRs is a quick and fairly simple process that can be done by any doctor who has been trained to understand and work with them. The corrections mostly involve very gentle cranial adjustments (making the small bones of the head and face move properly), freeing up the nerves so that they don't have to fire when they aren't supposed to, and adjusting the sacrum, or tailbone.

Most of the doctors in the United States whom I have trained to correct RPRs have been chiropractors at the vanguard of their profession, but there are also osteopaths and medical doctors who have learned these valuable tools for helping their patients. You can find a list of doctors across North America who are trained in RPR therapy by going to www.akcsm.com.

—James P. Blumenthal, DC, CCN, DACBN

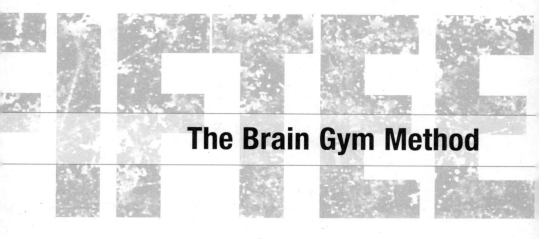

The Brain Gym Method

n today's high-stress world, more and more children are newly diagnosed with learning and/or behavior problems, which is a source of confusion, mystery, and sad frustration to parents. Labels abound: ADD, ADHD, dyslexia, autism, and so forth. Medications are often prescribed to handle the problems behind these labels; they may be necessary, but they are not sufficient on their own. Medications merely address symptoms, not root causes. The critical question that needs to be asked is this: Why do these children experience lack of focus, concentration, and myriad other symptoms?

Why do students daydream in class, failing to complete simple classroom assignments in time? Why do students have sloppy handwriting, and no matter how you try to motivate them to improve, they can't, or don't? It's deeply frustrating for parents and teachers, and for the students, too.

I've had these very same experiences with students in my twenty-five plus years of teaching. I knew there had to be a way to reach out and help these kids. The answers are not just about discipline; they are about how these children learn and why they can't.

That's exactly what motivated me to create Equilibrium—to find the solutions. I've observed several key factors. First, the key to eliminating the symptoms of ADD/ADHD and other problems is rooted in the physiology of the person—the brain-body connection.

Second, poor diet, overuse of antibiotics, and stress often play a far larger part in early learning patterns for kids than many of us realize. For example, erratic eating and erratic behaviors, abnormal fatigue, brain fog (which manifests as an inability to focus on or complete routine tasks), hypoglycemia, and even unrecognized candidiasis are some of the key causes and symptoms that need more effective intervention.

My research and testing resulted in the development of Equilibrium Integrative Brain Body Healing Techniques, creating drug-free ways of restoring balance and mental and physical clarity for myself and for kids and adults in need. Since shifting my focus away from classroom teaching, I have worked with clients with conditions labeled as ADD/ADHD, learning problems, dyslexia, autism, Down syndrome, and other special needs, including behavior issues, stress, self-esteem issues, and a host of other neurological disorders, even Lou Gehrig's disease and cerebral palsy.

Brain Gym is the foundation of my work. It consists of a series of specific movements that synchronize the brain and the body to reduce stress, improve learning, enhance creativity, and help people of all ages and types of challenges reach their personal goals. The twenty-six targeted movements address the physical skills of learning. When the neuropathways for movement are fired, they activate and connect the whole brain in the synergistic way necessary for growth and change. These safe and simple activities support people of any age with connecting to their full potential. The Brain Gym movements are a series of physical activities that create neural pathways and activate the brain and the rest of the body for particular skills of learning.

Brain Gym is part of an overall program called Educational Kinesiology or Edu-K. Kinesiology is the study of movement. According to the Brain Gym website, www.braingym.org, "Edu-K is the process of applying natural movement experiences to facilitate learning. Edu-K is a process for allowing the mind-body system to accomplish any skill or function with greater ease and efficiency."

Paul Dennison, an expert in the field of child motor development, and his wife, Gail Dennison, developed Brain Gym in the 1970s. He states that "movement is the door to learning." Brain Gym is moving the body to wake up the brain. Movement, learning, and brain development are all connected. Physical movement, from earliest infancy and throughout our lives, plays an important role in the creation of nerve cell networks, which are actually the essence of learning. The Brain Gym movements are simple activities that children do naturally in their first three years of development to accomplish important developmental steps for coordination of eyes, ears, hands, and the whole body.

The human brain has two hemispheres, the right and left, each with certain characteristics. The left brain deals with logic, sequence, and order; it sees the individual parts of a whole. The right brain deals with creativity, music, and art; it sees the whole picture. The goal for ease and efficiency in learning and other activities is to have whole brain learning with both hemispheres working together. At any age, when we experience stress, we lose access to whole brain connections. The nondominant side of the brain shuts down, and we can experience struggles in many areas. We enter survival mode, and we can't access the higher functions of the brain. Children may not be able to learn or behave with ease during these times.

Remember a situation when things went really well in your life. How did you feel? Did you have lots of energy, maybe great ideas, and feelings of happiness? This was whole brain integration. Now think of a situation that caused you a lot of stress. How did you feel? How was your energy level? Were you able to find new solutions to problems? Were you happy or frustrated? This is lack of whole brain integration.

As long as we are alive, we are always experiencing stress. How stressed do children feel when they are faced with learning or behavioral challenges and the labels thrust upon them?

Years ago, one of my first-grade students said, "I want to turn on the lights of my brain." With Brain Gym, we did. This child was headed for "special education" and a lifetime of struggle, failure, and low self-esteem. Instead, he was given the tools to succeed.

How do Brain Gym movements help us to achieve a whole brain state? The Brain Gym movements are grouped into four categories:

1. **Midline movements** address communication (the right and left hemispheres of the brain) and focus on the skills necessary for easy, two-sided movement across the midline of the body (left-right movements). They help integrate the functioning of both eyes together, both ears together, and the left and right sides of the brain and body.

2. **Energy exercises** help us with organization (the bottom and top of the brain) to reestablish the neural pathways between the brain and the rest of the body, thus facilitating the flow of electromagnetic energy throughout the body.

3. **Lengthening activities** address comprehension (the back and front of the brain) and help reset our proprioceptors—the brain cells in the muscles.

4. **Deepening attitudes** help us to deal with stress and move out of the fight or flight patterns and into the reasoning centers, allowing us to think and act.

With all of the Brain Gym movements, we can more easily communicate, focus, and organize our lives, learning and living. The Brain Gym gives people tools to improve their quality of life. When your brain and body are in balance, your life is in Equilibrium.

—Barbara Schwartz, MA, Integrative Healing Techniques Specialist

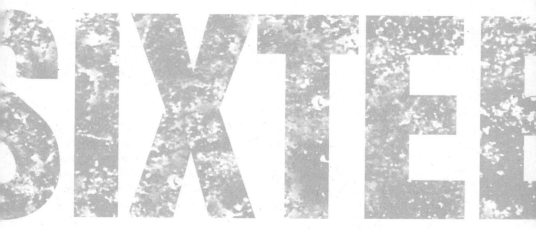

HEALING THE UNDERLYING EMOTIONAL
CONTRIBUTORS TO ADD AND ADHD

The three primary characteristics of ADD/ADHD are inattention, hyperactivity, and impulsivity. Each of these can be a function of a disruption of our body's energy system. Just as we have a circulatory system, a respiratory system, and a lymphatic system, our bodies are electromagnetic in nature and are run by our energy system.

Electroencephalography (EEG) is the measurement of electrical activity produced by the brain, and an electrocardiogram (ECG) is the measurement of the electrical activity of the heart over time. While Western medicine uses these tools, it hasn't yet recognized that our entire body and all of its organs and systems are connected to and dependent on our having a well-functioning electrical system consisting of our meridians, chakras, and our aura, or biofield.

The meridians were discovered and embraced by the Chinese over five thousand years ago. Since then, Traditional Chinese Medicine has recognized a subtle energy system by which chi (qi) is circulated through the body. When chi becomes blocked, the rest of the body that was being nourished by the continuous flow now suffers. Illness and disease can result if the flow is not restored.

It is becoming more and more apparent, with the convergence of science and spirituality, that thought processes and subconscious belief systems firmly entrenched in our bodies and energy systems cause or contribute to many of the challenges we humans encounter on a daily basis. Our emotional responses then release the powerful chemicals controlled by our brains and our hormones, which affect our bodies either positively or negatively. It has even been theorized that we can positively or negatively affect our genes! Although this has not yet become widely recognized by the medical community, some physicians and scientists have made breakthrough discoveries in what is now referred to as the science of epigenetics. According to Bruce H. Lipton, author of *The Biology of Belief*, "Recent advances in the science of epigenetics and quantum physics herald a global evolution that will profoundly impact the life of every person on this planet."

> I could see the terror on my friend Karen's face when we stopped at her house after she didn't show up at the beach. Through her fear she started laughing. "I really was going to come, but when I went to leave, my car had a flat tire . . . in my garage! I guess my fear of the water was strong enough to prevent me from going to the beach at any cost." She went on to explain that, although she had been a strong swimmer and even had her Senior Lifesaving certification, fifteen years ago she had been caught in a riptide and was dragged out far into the ocean and nearly drowned. Since then, it was difficult for her even to walk where the ocean meets the beach. We worked with Emotional Freedom Techniques for fifteen to twenty minutes on the fears and the incident that caused them—and her fear was gone. A fifteen-year phobia was gone that easily! The next day she bought a Boogie Board and a wetsuit. Her actions eventually lead to the formation of a group of ladies, all over fifty, who hang out on the beach at Del Mar, California, whom we lovingly refer to as the "Boogie Babes."

This is a very simple example of the power of a process called Emotional Freedom Techniques (EFT), one of a number of modalities falling under the heading of Energy Psychology. In Traditional Chinese Medicine, the use of acupuncture is common to balance the body's energy system. Instead of using needles, EFT uses a simple tapping method of two fingers on specific points of the body.

The three primary advantages of Emotional Freedom Techniques and Energy Medicine over psychiatric medications for ADD/ADHD are that they are non-invasive, highly specific, and have no side effects. The fourth advantage is that they have a very high rate of success. These methods balance the subtle energy systems of the body to help create peace, joy, and ease, physically, mentally, emotionally, and spiritually. They have been known to address almost any ailment known, mostly with a high rate of success. Symptoms of many chronic diseases have been mitigated or have even disappeared with the use of these simple methods.

In the span of one generation, we have discovered, or rediscovered, techniques that can make us happier, less stressed, and much healthier—safely, quickly, and without side effects. Techniques from Energy Medicine and Energy Psychology can alleviate chronic diseases, shift autoimmune conditions, and eliminate psychological traumas, with an efficiency and speed that conventional treatments can scarcely touch.

EFT is easily learned and can be easily applied to yourself or others. Children find it fun, and it makes them feel empowered because they are able to handle situations that may have previously been distressing to them. EFT helps to use our own natural energies to shift patterns of emotions, thoughts, and behaviors that are blatantly dysfunctional or merely self-limiting. I believe that all teachers should have instruction in EFT so that they can use it and teach it to their students. There is a saying among EFT practitioners: Try it on everything! One of the main results of EFT, regardless of what a person is working on, is a calm peacefulness, making it very effective for addressing the hyperactivity that often accompanies ADD. EFT can also help us to focus on a task at hand.

In my own practice, I focus on the emotional effect that the symptoms of a disturbance have on my client. This often leads to a core issue or the origin of the challenge that we are addressing. In the case of ADD/ADHD, my questions to my client would follow what complaints he reported. If he talked about being distracted at school, my first direction would be to ask how that made him feel. He might report that he felt frustrated by how distracted he gets. We would tap on the frustration along with tapping on the behavior that caused it. Initially I would have my client rate the level of distraction on a scale of zero to ten, zero meaning that he was able to be attentive and ten being the extreme of distraction. I would also ask him to rate the level of frustration that this was causing him. The tapping would have a beneficial effect on the three major symptoms of ADHD: hyperactivity, inattention, and impulsivity.

In the following paragraphs, we will be discussing what to say at the actual tapping points. You can download a free manual describing the process of EFT at www.emofree.com. You can also sign up for a free newsletter with wonderful tips on using EFT.

I would lead my client in the tapping process following the setup phrases. It might look something like this:

Tapping on the Karate Chop point (just below the side of the pinky finger on the fleshy side of your hand) with the tips of the fingers of the other hand and saying one of the following:

- "Even though I get really frustrated by getting so distracted in school, I still deeply and completely love and accept myself." (If working with a young child, we would say, "I'm still a good kid.")
- "Even though I hate having this ADD, I'm still a good kid."
- "Even though this frustration is as distracting as my ADD, I'm still a good kid."

Then, tapping on the EFT points, I usually use the two middle fingers of the other hand. It doesn't matter which hand you tap with or which side of the body you tap on:

LOCATION	ABBREVIATION	WHAT TO SAY
Beginning of eyebrow	EB	I'm really frustrated by this ADD.
Side of the eye	SE	I'm tired of being so distracted.
Under the eye (cheekbone)	UE	This frustration.
Under the nose	UN	I feel so frustrated.
Under the bottom lip (chin)	Ch	Why do I have to have ADD?
Under the collar bone	CB	Everybody seems to be frustrated with my ADD.
Under the arm (4 inches down)	UA	This frustration about ADD.
Top of head (crown)	TH	This frustration about being distracted.
Karate chop (below pinky)	KC	It's so hard to focus.
Inside of wrist (pulse point)	IW	I've been so impulsive I can't control it.
Back of the hand (between pinky finger bone and ring finger bone)	BH	I can't seem to relax.

When you have completed a round of tapping, notice any sensations in your body. Allow your body to give you a number between zero and ten that represents the level that the issue you were working on still feels like in your body. Then do another round of tapping. This round would use the same tapping points and the same statements.

As your distress levels are getting lower, you can tap in what it is that you want. Using the same tapping points, your statements would look like this:

LOCATION	WHAT TO SAY
EB	I choose to be calm and peaceful throughout my day.
SE	I relax, do my best, and life is beautiful.
UE	It's easy for me to keep my attention focused.
UN	I always think before I act.
Ch	My actions are appropriate to the situation.
CB	It is easy for me to remain focused and pay attention.
UA	I love myself exactly as I am.
TH	I choose to be calm and peaceful in all situations.
KC	My attention stays focused on what I am working on.
IW	I am grateful to release hyperactivity, inattention, and impulsivity.
BH	It's easy for me to focus.

You can continue alternating these until the level reaches zero.

This is the shortcut method. Download the complete seventy-nine-page manual at www.emofree.com. As I mentioned before, any time that you feel frustrated or have any negative emotion, pain, or stress, *tap on everything!*

Another major contributor to spectrum disorders is electromagnetic frequencies, or radiation. I call it Why Fry with WiFi?

Are we exposing ourselves and our children to dangerous electromagnetic radiation every day? More and more scientific studies are pointing in that direction.

Electromagnetic radiation is propagated through the atmosphere by broadcast towers, radar installations, satellite broadcasts, and microwave appliances. It is also generated by the magnetic fields surrounding cell phones, portable phones, electrical appliances, and power lines. I used to think you'd be safe in a cornfield in Iowa. But now, if you're lost in a cornfield, your electronic GPS, with its satellite transmissions, will help you find your way out!

Despite the fact that electropollution has been largely ignored in the United States, research indicates that it can cause extreme fatigue, insomnia, and depression and contributes to a vast number of other dangerous health effects including autism and ADHD. WiFi is now common in most U.S. coffeehouses and bookstores, and I even saw it in a local grocery store the other day. Last week a friend of mine came to my home, put her laptop on my dining room table, and connected to the Internet. I don't even have WiFi in my home! At an alarming rate, we are unknowingly exposing our children to this danger at home and in our schools.

Even more alarming is that the cellular industry is now aiming their advertising at the "tweeners," children between eight and twelve years of age. In George Carlo's book *Cell Phones: Invisible Hazards in the Wireless Age*, he quotes a study by Om Gandhi that found that the depth of penetration of the cell phone's damaging waves in a five-year-old's brain was over four times that of an adult. In a ten-year-old, the absorption rate is two and a half times that of an adult. My personal pet peeve is pregnant mothers who unknowingly carry a cell phone in their shoulder bag, right next to their baby's developing brain! Just as bad is when they are holding an infant or young child and are talking on their cell phone, unaware of the dangers.

But cell phones aren't the only problem. Think of the young men who grew up playing with video games. They held the remote controls on their laps while concentrating on the TV screen. Now they all have laptop computers that sit, where else, on their laps. And where do they carry their cell phones? In their pockets or on their belts. As a result, testicular cancer has increased by 50 percent in the last twenty years and infertility is on the rise.

Now, as in the past, one of the major concerns is about the radiation "plume" extending six to eight inches from the antenna of the cell phone. However, with the proliferation of electronics, the ambient energy in the atmosphere is now as dangerous as the plume of a cell phone. This is caused by high-wattage electrical devices, such as hair dryers and vacuum cleaners, cellular devices, portable phones (which are two to three times as dangerous as cell phones), and all of the satellites and transmission towers that serve them. What this means is that the exposure to electromagnetic radiation can be just as dangerous even if you don't use a cell phone or a computer!

A Swedish study warns specifically about the intense use of mobile phones by youngsters: The voluntary exposure of the brain to microwaves from hand-held mobile phones is "the largest human biological experiment ever." Leading experts are worried about the future of people's wellness. This newly recognized yet rapidly emerging toxin called electropollution may be silently accelerating the aging process, dangerously increasing stress levels, and preventing essential nutrients from entering the body's cells, as well as keeping damaging toxins from exiting the cells. The effect of electromagnetic radiation on our bodies has contributed to an increase in breast cancer, Alzheimer's, autism, ADD, and ADHD, just to name a few. In the '70s and '80s, autism was found in one in ten thousand children. It is now found in one in one hundred and fifty American children and about one in ninety-four boys.

Wireless technology is here to stay; this is the problem. Fortunately, there are solutions with proven technologies to limit exposure to all of these dangers. One of the most effective solutions is a cell chip developed by a Russian scientist. There are devices that put off waves that harmonize the potential damaging waves of electropollution.

Protect yourself and your family today so that you can *safely* enjoy all of the conveniences of these electronic devices.

—*Pat Farrell*

More Alternative
Approaches

159

What Is a Naturopathic Doctor?

aturopathic doctors (ND) are trained as primary care physicians who specialize in treating a variety of health conditions using natural therapies. They are considered to be a bridge between conventional and traditional medicine and have extensive experience treating patients suffering from ADHD and other neurological disorders.

After completing four years of postgraduate schooling at one of only six accredited naturopathic medical colleges in North America, naturopathic physicians must earn their board certification prior to becoming licensed to practice medicine.

The principles followed by naturopathic physicians are the following:

1. *Primum no nocere:* First, do no harm.
2. *Vis medicatrix naturae:* The healing power of nature.
3. *Tolle causum:* Identify and treat the cause.
4. *Tolle totem:* Treat the whole person.
5. *Docere:* Physician as teacher.
6. Prevention.

Depending upon the state in which an ND practices, some of these doctors are able to prescribe pharmaceutical drugs. However, naturopathic philosophy dictates that natural, holistic treatments be initially used. These treatments include the use of herbs, nutrients, homeopathic remedies, dietary changes, physical medicine, and hydrotherapy, just to name a few.

The treatment chosen depends entirely on the individual's health status along with his or her current health challenges. Many chronic conditions unresponsive to conventional (allopathic) therapies often fare well when treated with naturopathic therapeutics.

The healing approach of an ND involves determining a "cause" for a specific illness and then treating or removing that cause, as opposed to merely masking symptoms with medication. These well-trained doctors use standard testing methods, such as X-rays, blood tests, physical exams, ultrasound, and other diagnostic techniques to arrive at the "cause" of a patient's illness. Once this "obstacle to cure" has been removed, optimal wellness may be achieved. This approach can be used to treat illnesses ranging from allergies and asthma to heart disease and cancers.

A naturopathic physician uses this approach in treating ADHD and other autism spectrum disorders (ASD). The approach begins with ordering diagnostic tests, which might include obtaining stool samples to determine the presence of yeast overgrowth, standard blood tests to determine the overall health and nutritional status of the patient, and organic amino acid tests. Once a "cause" has been established, an individualized treatment plan is developed to help remove the "cause" using herbs, nutrients, dietary modifications, or homeopathic remedies. In the case of ADHD, the culprit is often determined to be a food sensitivity or sensitivity to a particular preservative or food dye. By removing the offending item, many children diagnosed with ADHD notice marked improvement in their behavior.

When treating children with autism, NDs often incorporate therapies that support the child's immune system. This might include restoring their digestion by eliminating yeast overgrowth, giving them homeopathic remedies that help antidote adverse reactions to vaccines, and prescribing supplements to improve their nutritional status.

A therapy that is often used when treating ADHD and ASD is called craniosacral therapy. This hands-on treatment was developed by an osteopathic physician.

During a craniosacral therapy session, the patient lies fully clothed on his or her back while the practitioner uses a series of gentle maneuvers to help restore balance to the lymphatic system. After a few moments, the patient enters a state of relaxation caused by a natural parasympathetic response of the body to this hands-on technique. The parasympathetic nervous system is a division of the autonomic nervous system, and it is responsible for promoting a restful state, in addition to promoting digestion. Its counterpart is the sympathetic nervous system, which is responsible for causing a "fight or flight" response. So it is easy to see how invoking a restful state would be beneficial when treating ADHD and ASD. But craniosacral therapy goes well beyond merely invoking a parasympathetic state. It also assists in removing blockages throughout the body. Many practitioners believe that the combined effects of craniosacral therapy serve as a useful adjunct to other naturopathic treatments for ADHD/ASD.

As you can see, naturopathic physicians utilize a wide variety of treatment modalities when considering various health challenges. It is this approach, along with their respect for a mind-body connection in medicine, that sets this profession apart from other health care practitioners.

—Lesa Werner, ND

Homeopathy and ADHD

ttention deficit hyperactivity disorder is a diagnosis given to 10 percent of all school children in America. In 1985, five hundred thousand children in the United States were diagnosed with ADHD. Today there are between five and seven million. In a class with thirty children, between one and three children are diagnosed with ADHD.

Often parents have an idea that their child may have emotional or behavioral problems because of an erratic behavior. They might have assumed that this was simply their child's kinetic personality coupled with a developing young mind. ADHD is a neurobehavioral disorder associated with difficulty in learning and concentration, inattentive behavior, impulsiveness, and emotional problems.

The medical community informs parents that the only way to eradicate the symptoms is by using medication. Most of these medications are stimulants, which have the effect of refining focus of thought so that the child can attend to school and homework and not be a disturbance in the classroom. Perhaps some parents are elated to know that there is a medicine to cure the problem. However, all drugs have side effects. Ritalin has been associated with sleeplessness, addiction, depression, and other unpleasant consequences. At the beginning of the treatment, the side effects can be quite serious. Besides changing the child's behavior from unruliness to docility, making him more socially acceptable, Ritalin can cause nausea, vomiting, mood swings, loss of appetite, decreased height, and weight loss.

Due to the drug's many side effects, some parents look for alternative ways to help their suffering children. Prompted by their desire to find the best solution for the child, some families find their way to homeopathy.

What Is Homeopathy?

Homeopathy is essentially an energetic treatment method based on the fact that matter and energy are the same, existing in different forms and subject to change. Homeopathic remedies help to exert a positive constitutional change, and the results are possibly due to unobserved quantum effects. The homeopathic system is based on the principle that diseases can be cured with minute doses of drugs, which in a healthy person in large doses would produce symptoms like those of the disease.

You may have treated yourself homeopathically when you were ill and took a substance that produces in a healthy person the symptoms of your illness. For example, in many cultures raw onion and garlic are used to treat colds. A cut onion may make our eyes and nose run with burning discharges and causes us to sneeze. These are the same symptoms we have with a cold. In some ways, homeopathy can be compared to a vaccination. However, vaccines are live viruses or bacteria. In addition, if you receive quinine for malaria, colchicine for gout, or radiation for skin cancer, you are being treated with a remedy that could produce the symptoms of your ailment in a healthy person. Homeopathic remedies have no trace of a mother tincture left. The remedy is so highly diluted that it is called an "imprint" of the substance used.

Homeopathy has been practiced for two hundred years and is not a new treatment method or medical craze. My grandparents saw only homeopaths for their health issues. My parents, however, went to medical doctors first, often with unsatisfactory results. Inevitably, they too went to the homeopath. Most often, my parents resorted to homeopathic remedies and herbs to cure everything from colds to childhood diseases.

How Are Homeopathic Medicines Produced?

Homeopathic medicines are dilutions prepared from many natural substances, mainly herbs. But there are also remedies prepared from animal and bacterial tissues. The remedies are made by successive dilutions, meaning they are diluted with water, then a drop from the dilution is again mixed with a certain amount of water, and so on. At each step of dilution, the substance is shaken (succussed) a number of times to reach the desired potency. The more the remedy is diluted, the more powerful it becomes; it is not understood why, but theories are being tested and a greater understanding is inevitable. In the meantime, we know that homeopathy works as "energy" medicine.

Why Is Homeopathy So Effective?

The reason homeopathy is so effective is that it treats the whole person and not the disease. The treatment is not based on ICD9 codes (international statistical classifications of diseases and related health problems). Homeopaths do not diagnose. Rather, they prescribe remedies based on a symptom picture given by the patient, including all aches and pains from head to toe. This includes the mind, the emotions, and the time of day when conditions are worse, too cold, or too hot. Subjective symptoms are very important. They are often private and secret feelings, but when they are expressed, they become vital clues for determining a remedy.

Homeopathy for Attention Deficit Disorder

Based on the method in which homeopathy is used, it can be a powerful tool to treat troubled children as well as adults suffering from ADHD and other behavioral disorders. As a first aid, homeopathy can treat sleeplessness, anxiety, nervousness, and hyperactivity. An overly impulsive child can be helped with a remedy that makes him stop to think first and act later. For example, there is Coffea cruda, which is coffee. When given in a microdose, coffee is used for sleeplessness. Chamomile is used for the hyperactive child. Arsenicum Album and Argentum Nitricum are used for anxiety and with those who suffer from fears. It is advisable not to change remedies too often. Let one bring about the desired result first. Sometimes one remedy acts for a long time.

Since ADHD displays a myriad of symptoms and every person has his or her own unique biochemical makeup, it is recommended to seek the help of an experienced homeopathic practitioner. Parents should inform themselves about homeopathic medicines before they use any, and the remedies should only be used as first aid. A homeopath should be considered for constitutional treatments.

How Can I Find the Correct Homeopathic Remedy?

The correct remedy is found by checking a multitude of symptoms against a multitude of remedies in what is called the homeopathic repertory and homeopathic materia medica. It takes a lot of skill and expertise on the part of the practitioner to find the correct medicine. But when it is found, it works like a miracle. It happens sometimes that the practitioner has to try several remedies or several different potencies for the patient to achieve the desired state of health, but when the correct remedy is found, the result can be instantaneous.

Homeopathic Medicines Are Catalysts

Homeopathic medicines work together with our own healing powers. Our bodies are equipped to heal themselves when nutritional conditions are homeostatic. Many times we may feel ill one day, thinking something is "coming on," and the next day we are fine again; the body has taken care of it overnight. Sometimes this ideal condition breaks down and we get sick. Our weakened vital force cannot handle the attack and needs help. The help comes in a well-chosen homeopathic remedy that is based on the patient's symptoms. It will give the body's vital force the desired push toward health. Many times the remedies work profoundly by eliminating long-standing, chronic illnesses in a process that can be compared to a deep spring-cleaning of the body. With well-chosen medicines, symptoms disappear from the inside out, from above downward, from more important organs to less important organs, and finally, from the extremities upward. Your feelings of fear and anxiety and other negative emotions are also swept away in this deep cleaning process. The patient emerges stronger in body, mind, and spirit.

Does Homeopathy Interfere with Other Medicines?

Homeopathy is gentle and harmless. It does not interfere with any other mode of treatment. You can treat yourself and your children while saving a lot of money. Remedy kits with first aid medicines are available at low cost. These are easy-to-take, small, sweet pellets or tablets. It is best to take them on their own, not with food or drink, preferably at bedtime. Remedies last for a long time and don't lose their effectiveness. They should be stored away from extreme temperatures and strong-smelling chemicals and substances, like perfume.

Protocol for Taking Homeopathic Medicine

Without touching the tablets or pellets, shake four to six of them into the cap that covers the bottle. Put them under your tongue and let them dissolve. Don't eat or drink anything twenty minutes before or after taking them. Make sure your mouth is free of flavors like mint, coffee, or anything with a strong taste. The medicine is best taken at bedtime, but any time is equally good if the above precautions are observed.

Always Consult a Homeopathic Professional

Be aware that homeopathy is a serious medical specialty, and although I've portrayed it here simplistically for home use, individuals should never attempt to treat constitutional or life-threatening illnesses. A constitutional illness is a health problem of long standing or a chronic condition that a person is born with or has inherited tendencies toward. Any condition that does not show quick improvement must be referred to a qualified practitioner or medical doctor, preferably a medical doctor who specializes in homeopathy. Besides, nothing is more difficult for a homeopathic practitioner to unravel than a case of unsuccessful self-treatments with partially indicated remedies. It is advised to always consult with your child's medical doctor before attempting a new treatment.

—Marlene McKee, NE, DIHom

CHAPTER 19

Adverse Reactions to Ritalin and Other Medications

Warning: Never discontinue taking stimulants or antidepressants without first consulting your health care professional. The withdrawal symptoms can be more severe than the adverse reactions to these medications; therefore, the process must be closely monitored by a mental health professional.

To medicate or not to medicate. This was the center of family discussions while my kids were in elementary school. Many teachers, doctors, psychologists, friends, and family members were strongly recommending that we put both Erik and Westley on stimulants. My husband said he wouldn't allow our children to take speed. At this time, I was only aware of a few potential side effects, such as suppressed appetite, insomnia, and symptoms of Tourette's syndrome. I was opposed to my kids being medicated; they were only in the tenth to twenty-fifth percentile for their height and weight, and Westley was exhibiting some facial tics. I was no expert on ADHD or medication, but I knew that sleep is critical for producing human growth hormone and that children need to eat to grow. It seemed to me that the effects of Ritalin would conflict with what is natural for a healthy, growing body. There is no drug that can cure ADHD. The drugs may suppress some of the symptoms, but not without many potentially serious side effects, and ADHD drugs are prescribed for long-term use.

I know one boy who suffered depression and hallucinations while taking Ritalin. He stopped taking the medication after using it for seven years. When asked how he felt while taking Ritalin, he described it as always feeling depressed. He would be hungry, but he wouldn't eat much. He would feel tired, but he couldn't fall asleep. He felt like his energy was stuck inside his body, but he was unable to express it. Once he was off the drug, he felt much better.

Witnessing the side effects this boy experienced made me that much more determined to discover natural, alternative solutions.

Facts about Ritalin and Other Medications Used to Treat ADD/ADHD

- The government estimates that 2.5 million American children and 1.5 million American adults take medication for ADHD.

- The side effects reported on Ritalin's label include stomachaches, headaches, and hallucinations, but reports have suggested it also causes more severe reactions, such as liver problems and even death. The FDA's advisory committee voted eight to seven in favor of putting a black box warning—the FDA's most severe warning for side effects in drugs—on the box of Ritalin, but the FDA has not yet taken any action on the recommendation. This was after data revealed that ADHD drugs may have caused twenty-five deaths and fifty-four serious medical problems among patients between the years 1999 and 2003. Cited medical problems include stroke, hypertension, palpitations, arrhythmia, and heart attacks.

- Between the years 1990 and 2000, more than 569 children were hospitalized—thirty-eight of them were life-threatening hospitalizations—and 186 died, all from using stimulants. Many of them died from cardiac arrest and strokes.

- All stimulants cause constriction of veins and arteries, causing the heart to work overtime, leading to damage to the heart.

- Victoria Vetter, a pediatric cardiologist at the University of Pennsylvania School of Medicine and the head of the heart group committee, recommends that children should have an EKG to rule out any undiagnosed heart issues before they are put on drugs. She said that after screening 1,100 children she found that fully 2 percent of them had some kind of heart problem.

- Schools receive additional money from the state and federal governments for every child labeled and drugged.

- Children twelve years and older who have been prescribed or are currently taking any stimulants or antidepressants are automatically rejected for military service.

- Amphetamines like Dexedrine and Adderall are toxic to the brain and can cause brain cell death. In several studies with lab animals, such as rhesus monkeys, small doses of amphetamines were administered over periods of days or weeks. The animals showed a lasting loss of receptors for the neurotransmitter dopamine.

- Ritalin is highly addictive. It's a Schedule II category drug, along with morphine, cocaine, opium, and barbiturates. The common street names for Ritalin include rids, pineapple, and kiddie cocaine.

- No studies have been conducted on Ritalin for children under six years old.

- Strattera is the newest drug that Eli Lilly & Company is promoting for ADHD. It's been dispensed to more than two million patients since it went on the market in 2002. Eli Lilly & Company was required to include a black box warning on the package stating the following:

> Even though there has not been a direct link established between violent crimes and taking prescription antidepressants and stimulants, the most tragic cases of violent murder by someone on prescription drugs should be noted.

- Jeffrey Weiss went on a shooting rampage on March 21, 2005, at Red Lake High School that left ten dead, including him. Earlier that day, Weiss had killed his grandfather and his grandfather's girlfriend. He was on Prozac and recently the dosage had been increased.

- Eric Harris, one of the killers at Columbine High School, was on the antidepressant drug Luvox. Court records show that the prescription for Harris had been filled ten times between April 1998 and March 1999. Three and a half months before the shooting, the dosage had been increased. The *Physician's Desk Reference* records show that during controlled clinical trials of Luvox, manic reactions developed in 4 percent of the children given the drug.

- Thomas Solomon, a fifteen-year-old at Heritage High School in Conyers, Georgia, shot and wounded six classmates. He was on Ritalin at the time.

SAFETY INFORMATION

In some children and teens, Strattera increases the risk of suicidal thoughts. A combined analysis of twelve studies of Strattera showed that in children and teens this risk was 0.4 percent for those taking Strattera compared to none for those taking a sugar pill. A similar analysis in adults treated with Strattera did not reveal an increased risk of suicidal thoughts. Call your doctor right away if your child has thoughts of suicide or sudden changes in mood or behavior, especially at the beginning of treatment or after a change in dose.

- Kip Kinkel, a fifteen-year-old at Thurston High School in Springfield, Oregon, killed his parents and two classmates and wounded twenty-two other students while on Ritalin and Prozac.

- Shawn Cooper, a fifteen-year-old sophomore at Notus Junior-Senior High School in Notus, Idaho, fired a shotgun at his fellow students. He was on Ritalin.

- In 1989, less than one month after taking his first dose of Prozac, Joseph Wesbecker massacred eight coworkers with an AK-47 before turning the weapon on himself.

- Michael McDermott, convicted of killing seven co-workers, tripled his dosage of Prozac before the shootings. On the witness stand he said he believed that he killed Nazis and not his co-workers. He said an archangel appeared to him before the massacre, telling him that he could prevent the Holocaust if he traveled back in time to 1940 to kill Adolf Hitler and six German generals.

- Brynn Hartman, wife of comedian Phil Hartman, shot and killed her husband and herself while on Zoloft.

- Andrea Yates in Houston, Texas, drowned her five children while on Effexor and Remeron.

- Christopher Pittman shot and killed his grandparents when he was age twelve. He claimed that a voice inside his head told him to kill his grandparents on November 28, 2001. Christopher had recently started to take Zoloft to treat mild depression.

—Deborah Merlin

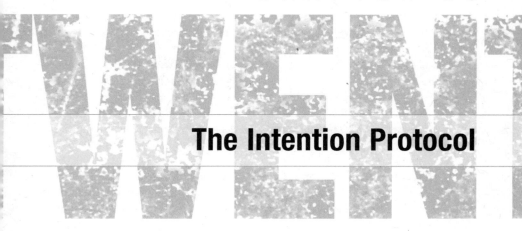

The Intention Protocol

Parents, you have been given valuable information to enable you to find the best approaches to help your child. All the treatments previously described in this book assist the physiology of the body to move toward balance.

There is one other treatment modality that can be used in combination with all the others described in this book. This treatment modality involves using the power of your intention. Your conscious intention combined with your love for your child unites into a powerful force. In this section we will discuss how intention works and give you a protocol for setting intention to create the best possible outcomes for your child.

First, it helps to know something about the playing field—the quantum field. When you were in school you probably saw diagrams of atoms as the building blocks of matter, with electrons depicted as tiny little balls spinning around the central core of the atom. The truth is that the electrons move around the nucleus of the atom as fields of probability. Scientists can't even measure an electron's position and its velocity (speed and direction) at the same time. If they measure the electron's position, the act of measuring affects the electron's velocity in unpredictable ways. If they measure the velocity, the act of measuring disrupts the electron's position. This inability to measure a particle's position and velocity simultaneously is called the uncertainty principle. The uncertainty principle applies to any subatomic particle, such as photons and quarks, and is the first step in understanding that matter is affected by intention. These particles dance in and out of existence in and around us, creating the quantum field. They can manifest as waves or particles. Think of the wave nature as a plucked and vibrating guitar string.

Experiments (such as the double-slit experiment) have shown that the act of observation of subatomic particles and the observer's expectations determine which form will manifest. This is known as the observer effect.

It was thought until recently that these quantum effects only applied to the subatomic level, not to the molecular level. A team in Vienna repeated the double-slit experiment using large molecules, which consist of groups of atoms. The team had the same result as the double-slit experiment. So, these quantum observer effects occur in the realm of the everyday, not just in the subatomic realm. Matter can change form depending on what we expect to see, and therefore it is malleable to human intention and expectation.

If you're amazed by the observer effect, the idea of nonlocality will knock your socks off. A local effect is one that travels directly and continuously through time and space. A bowling ball hitting a pin is an example of a local effect. A radio signal from a transmitter tower picked up by your cell phone is another example of a direct or local effect. It takes time for the effect to occur and the movement is continuous throughout space. Nonlocality means that the effect is not transmitted through time and space. It is instantaneous and occurs without a specific signal traveling through space. Nonlocality was demonstrated initially in 1982 when lasers were used to heat calcium atoms. When calcium atoms are heated they give off pairs of photons, which bend light in a specific way. Because these photon pairs were created at the exact same moment from the same atom, they are said to be "entangled." The scientists then separated the photons and observed them. Even after the twin photons were separated, they still moved in unison. It wasn't possible for there to be any kind of direct effect between them; they were separated in space and the action was instantaneous. So, the effect is a quantum effect.

Any objects (or people) that have had a connection can have communication that is beyond space and time. This is called action at a distance; it is what Einstein called spooky. I call it an opportunity to recognize that the fundamental laws of our universe, of all matter, appear to be magical—until we understand the science behind them.

The principle of nonlocality is such an important one for us to grasp; it is the foundation for understanding how intention works. Any two particles in the universe that have been connected in some way can have a nonlocal relationship and are said to be entangled. You and your child have a local and a nonlocal relationship, and you definitely are "entangled." Although you appear solid and separate, both of you are composed of quantum fields of probabilities that can be affected by thoughts and feelings instantaneously at a distance.

Hundreds of experiments have been performed that have demonstrated the ability of individuals to effect changes at a distance in machines, plants, and people. In her book *The Intention Experiment*, Lynne McTaggart writes about a study in which a researcher asked two people to meditate together until they felt some kind of communication with each other. Then they entered separate rooms. Both participants were connected to EEG machines to measure their brain waves. One of them was shown a flickering light subliminally, so that on a conscious level he wasn't aware of it. The light signal produced a response in his brain, which looked like a spike on the graph paper. The partner in the other room simultaneously showed a similar spike in his EEG. Neither person knew what was being done to them beyond the fact that they were supposed to meditate and create a connection. From a quantum perspective, the two people were like twinned photons that were entangled and therefore could create a nonlocal effect.

This action at a distance has been demonstrated in many experiments with healing. For example, William Braud and his colleagues conducted experiments during which changes in physiological responses, such as blood pressure, were intended by senders and demonstrated in receivers. The results over seventeen years of experiments were found to be highly statistically significant. The possibility of the results being due to chance was calculated at more than a hundred trillion to one.

Now let's look at how you, a twinned pair with your child, can create nonlocal effects.

Intention Protocol

1. Sit where you will not be interrupted. Close your eyes and do some deep breathing. Focus in your mind's eye on something that makes you smile, makes you feel warm and fuzzy inside, or makes you feel at peace. It could be a shared moment of love, the way you feel in nature, or a sense of gratitude. Feel this love, peacefulness, or gratitude in your heart. Practice being able to bring it on at will. Although many scientific experiments have shown positive results simply by using intention, in my experience love provides the power and the intention provides the focus for that power.

2. Invite your child into your awareness. You may do so by picturing your child in your mind's eye or inviting your child into your heart space. Maintain the positive feeling. State your intention. The more specific, the better. Examples include statements such as "My child follows the teacher's instructions well in class," or "The neurons in my child's brain function perfectly," or "I see my child looking relaxed and happy." Hold that positive feeling as you see, feel, and know this is so. Be aware of any positive images, words, or ideas that occur to you. You may want to keep a journal of these impressions.

   Remember that when you are in this positive state, you also are in a state of fulfillment. Avoid being in a state of "wanting" or "needing" or "hoping" while doing the Intention Protocol. Experience the feeling of the end result in the present moment.

3. Let go of the need for results. You must release any need to help your child or to make things happen. Remember this is not a local effect. You cannot push to make something happen using the Intention Protocol. Be specific about your intention, but don't be too specific about the way in

which it occurs. When you allow your intention to manifest in its own way, you are making a space for synchronicity.

4. Hold the image and feeling for as long as it is comfortable to do so. Recreate that feeling and intention daily. Recognize that change may take place instantaneously or play out over time. Hold the feeling of anticipation and expectation that new information, assistance, and changes are around each corner.

Consider how many emotionally charged experiences your child has in a day. It may be his or her frustration with school or peers, your anger or frustration at him or her, or something else. Sometimes parents find the challenges of taking care of their child's physical needs so exhausting that they lose some of the joy of being a parent and having a special bond with their child. If it's been a tough day for both of you, don't berate yourself. Simply take time as soon as you can to envelop your child in this positive field of love and intention. It's great to do at night after your child goes to sleep.

The Intention Protocol provides you with a way to recapture the emotional rewards of being a parent. You will find that your own stress level will decrease, which in turn will affect your child and your child's interactions with others in a positive way. Remember that this is meant to be an enjoyable process, not hard work! Allow the Intention Protocol to help you to find the joy again in your life and in your relationship with your child.

—Kathleen Lewis, DC

Tests and Testing Laboratories

Your pediatrician or other doctors may not be familiar with these tests. The laboratory personnel can consult with your doctor or can provide names of doctors closest to your area who have knowledge of these tests and thereby provide proper guidance in treating your child. Most of the tests listed are covered by insurance.

Types of Tests

Food and inhalant allergy testing. Children with ADHD and autism often have food allergies, and symptoms worsen after the children eat certain foods. Candidiasis (yeast overgrowth) contributes to food allergies. IgG testing shows delayed food sensitivities.

Amino acid deficiencies. Amino acids are the basic building blocks of protein. They form neurotransmitters in the brain that regulate mood and behavior.

Candidiasis. Candidiasis is an overgrowth of yeast and may lead to leaky gut syndrome. Many ADHD and autistic children have tested positive for abnormally high levels of yeast. Gastrointestinal health panel (GI panel) and comprehensive digestive stool analysis (CDSA) are good tests for specific measures of intestinal health that can give rise to yeast, pathogenic bacteria, and parasite overgrowths.

Digestive function. People with autism and ADHD often exhibit chronic digestive problems. The GI panel and CDSA provide the best information to lead to treatment for digestive disorders. Poor digestion can result from an overuse of antibiotics.

Essential fatty acids. Deficiencies in essential fatty acids are very common among children with ADHD.

Heavy metal analysis. People with ADD/ADHD typically do very well once toxic metals are removed from the body. Urine tests are the most reliable and easiest method to check for heavy metals. Hair testing was popular at one time, but because hair is usually contaminated by cosmetics (such as shampoos) and the environment, it is not an accurate or reliable measurement.

Pesticides and flame-retardant chemicals. All individuals who have symptoms of ADHD, autism, learning disabilities, convulsions, chronic pain, and/or poor coordination should be checked for toxic chemical exposure. This is one of the most overlooked and potentially most important areas of concern because it has a direct and major effect on brain and body chemistry, is a serious problem for a large number of people, and is relatively easy to correct once the details are known.

Seizures. It is estimated that up to 38 percent of children diagnosed with ADHD have underlying seizures. A higher than usual incidence of seizures is seen in children with autism and Tourette's syndrome. Testing for amino acids, essential fatty acids, food allergies, environmental toxins, and heavy metals are important for assessing the causes and potential treatment of seizures.

Zinc testing and nutritional testing. Zinc and nutritional deficiencies are common in people with ADD/ADHD.

Testing Resources

Diagnos-Techs, Inc.
Clinical and Research Laboratory

6620 S. 192nd Place, Building J   www.diagnostechs.com
Kent, WA 98032   800-878-3787

Tests and services: gastrointestinal health panel

Doctor's Data, Inc.

3755 Illinois Avenue   www.doctorsdata.com
St. Charles, IL 60174-2420   800-323-2784

Tests and services: urine toxic and essential elements; fecal metals; comprehensive drinking water analysis; yeast culture and sensitivities

Environmental Health Center

8345 Walnut Hill Lane, Suite 200   www.ehcd.com
Dallas, TX 75231   214-368-4132

Tests and services: complete blood lab; comprehensive allergy and chemical testing; antigen lab; detoxification sauna; exercise facility; nutritional counseling and education; sauna and massage; environmentally safe facility; purified air and water; toxicological profiles

Genova Diagnostics

63 Zillicoa Street   www.genovadiagnostics.com
Asheville, North Carolina 28801   800-522-4762

Tests and services: genetic testing for problems with detoxification pathways; consultations regarding the decision to vaccinate; polypeptide; organic acids; digestive function; intestinal permeability

The Great Plains Laboratory, Inc.

11813 W. 77th Street   www.greatplainslaboratory.com
Lenexa, KS 66214   913-341-8949

Tests and services: organic acid test for yeast and bacteria overgrowth; vitamin and mineral deficiencies; opiate peptides for gluten and casein sensitivity; toxic exposures to heavy metals; deficiencies in the immune system; abnormal amino acid; comprehensive stool testing

Metametrix Clinical Laboratory

3425 Corporate Way
Duluth, GA 30096

www.metametrix.com
800-221-4640

Tests and services: fatty acids; amino acid profiles; IgE and IgG food antibodies; inhalant antibodies; organic acids test

Neurogistics, Inc.
Balance Your Child's Brain

876 Loop 337, Suite 305
New Braunfels, TX 78130

www.balanceyourchildsbrain.com
888-257-9068

Tests and services: neurotransmitter testing; neurotransmitter counseling; psychoeducation programs and counseling; customized protocols; supplementation; follow-up program

Pain and Stress Center

5282 Medical Drive #160
San Antonio, TX 78229-5379

www.painstresscenter.com
800-669-2256

Tests and services: nutritional counseling; amino acid testing; food allergy testing; orthomolecular programs; group lectures; educational programs; product research and development; amino acid supplements (call for catalog)

US Biotek Laboratories

13500 Linden Avenue North
Seattle, WA 98133

www.usbiotek.com
877-318-8728

Tests and services: serum IgG and IgE antibody panels for foods, indoor/outdoor inhalants, spices and herbs; serum or finger stick IgG antibody panels for foods, indoor/outdoor inhalants, spices and herbs; *Candida* antibodies; serum or finger stick IgG, A, M, and *Candida* antigen; comprehensive urinary metabolic profile (GC/MS); environmental pollutants panel (GC/MS); high-sensitivity CRP (hs-CRP)

Q-Metrx Inc. (QEEG)

1612 W. Olive Avenue, Suite 301
Burbank, CA 91506

www.q-metrx.com
818-563-5409

Tests and services: provides QEEG services nationally and internationally; accepts digital EEGs sent through the Internet for expert analysis and interpretation

Resources

Clinic

The HANDLE Institute

1300 Dexter Avenue North
110 The Casey Family Building
Seattle, WA 98109

www.handle.org
206-204-6000

The HANDLE Institute provides an effective, nondrug alternative for identifying and treating most neurodevelopmental disorders across the lifespan, including autism, ADD, ADHD, dyslexia, and Tourette's syndrome.

DVD

Autism, The Misdiagnosis of Our Future Generations by Dr. Buttar is available from www.TheMedicalSeries.com.

Household Lead Testing Kits

www.leadcheck.com
800-262-5323

Mercury-Free Dentist Referral Service

International Academy of Oral Medicine and Toxicology

www.iaomt.org
863-420-6373

Naturopathic Physician Locator

The American Association of Naturopathic Physicians

www.naturopathic.org

Magazines and Newsletters

Alternative Medicine
Mothering Magazine

www.alternativemedicine.com
www.mothering.com

Supplements

Child Life Essentials

4051 Glencoe Avenue, Suite 11
Marina Del Rey, CA 90292

www.childlife.net
800-993-0332

Nutritional supplements for children and infants.

Craig Nutraceuticals, Inc. (CNI)

3075 Alhambra Drive, Suite 206   www.cni-web.com
Cameron Park, CA 95682   800-293-1683

Amino acid and nutritional supplements.

Metabolic Maintenance Products

68994 N. Pine Street   www.metabolicmaintenance.com
Sisters, OR 97759   800-772-7873

Customized amino acid formula based on your amino acid profile from any reputable testing laboratory.

Springboard

3115 Stoney Oak Drive   www.SB3.com
Spring Valley, CA 91978   800-662-8045

Advanced transdermal cream, amino acid, and nutritional supplements.

Detoxification Products

The American Botanical Pharmacy

4114 Glencoe Avenue   www.herbdoc.com
Marina Del Rey, CA 90292   800-437-2362

Dr. Schultz Superfood and intestinal, liver, and gallbladder detoxification herbal formulas.

BioRay, Inc.

23151 Alcalde Drive, Suite C-3   www.Bioray2000.com
Laguna Hills, CA 92653   888-635-9582

Organic dietary supplement for detoxification of heavy metals and chemicals.

CompliMed

www.complimed.com   800-261-7276

Homeopathic medicine detoxification for environmental chemical/pesticide toxins and allergies.

Renew Life

www.renewlife.com   1-800-830-1800

Cleansing products for candidiasis and heavy metals.

Websites

www.bluedominoes.com   www.healthynewsletter.com
www.ethicsinmedicine.us   www.mercola.com
www.healthychild.com   www.naturalnews.com
www.sarnet.org

Recommended Products

(available in major health food stores and homeopathic pharmacies)

Digestive Flora

Promotes nutrient absorption, reduces food sensitivity, boosts immune function, rids the body of pathogens that can upset nutrient absorption, enhances digestive tract integrity and respiratory health, and facilitates better liver function, detoxification, and proper elimination.

Bio-K+   www.biokplus.com

Enterogenic Concentrate   www.professionalsupplementcenter.com
from Tyler Encapsulation

Jarro-dophilus EPS   www.jarrow.com
from Jarrow Formulas

Electromagnetic Protection Products

BIOPRO Technology   www.mybiopro.com/patfarrell

760-961-4027

Chips for cell phones and computers. Products to harmonize the electromagnetic frequencies in your home and protect you from EMFs in the ambient energy outside. Nutrition products to repair damage done to your body by EMFs.

Essential Fatty Acids

The following fish oils are all certified as containing no heavy metals.

Carlson Nutritional Supplements   www.carlsonlabs.com

Health from the Sun   www.healthfromthesun.com

Nordic Naturals   www.nordicnaturals.com

Flaxseed Oil

Barlean's Organic Oils   www.barleans.com

Spectrum Essentials   www.spectrumorganics.com

Udo's Choice   www.udoerasmus.com

Minerals

Trace Mineral Research　　　　www.traceminerals.com

Homeopathic Products for ADHD and Related Symptoms

Dr. Garber's Natural Solutions　　　　www.drgarbers.com

Homeopathic biotherapy formulas for anxiety, allergies, depression, constipation, sleeplessness, and other conditions.

Hyland's　　　　www.hylands.com

Calm Forté 4 Kids is a mild, nonaddictive, homeopathic remedy for promoting comfortable relaxation.

Lead-Free Art Supplies

bluedominoes, inc.　　　　www.bluedominoes.com

Creates and markets children's lead-free art supplies using only food grade ingredients and responsibly tests all ingredients and packaging for harmful substances.

References

SECTION II
FOOD COLORING, TOXIC METALS, AND ASPARTAME

Artificial Food and Cosmetic Coloring: A Hidden Source of Toxic Metals

California Department of Public Health, Childhood Lead Poisoning Prevention Branch. http://www.dhs.ca.gov/childlead/tableware/twinfo.html.

California Environmental Protection Agency Office of Environmental Health Hazard Assessment. 2006. "Development of Health Criteria for School Site Risk Assessment Pursuant to Health and Safety Code Section 901(g): Proposed Child Specific Benchmark Change in Blood Lead Concentration for School Site Risk Assessment." *Ca. Gov.* http://www.oehha.ca.gov/public_info/public/kids/pdf/PbHGV44_010507.pdf.

Contra Costa County Lead Poisoning Prevention Project. http://www.cchealth.org/topics/lead_poison/pdf/ceramics.pdf.

Haas, Elson, and Buck Levin. 2006. *Staying Healthy with Nutrition: The Complete Guide to Diet and Nutritional Medicine*. Berkeley, CA: Celestial Arts.

Hallaway, Nancy, and Zigurts Strauts. 1995. *Turning Lead into Gold: How Heavy Metal Poisoning Can Affect Your Child and How to Prevent and Treat It*. Vancouver, BC: New Star Books.

Kansas State University. 1995. "FDA Samples for Lead in Tableware." *Foods and Nutrition Digest*. http://www.oznet.k-state.edu/humannutrition/_fndigest/1995/mayjun95.htm#t3.

Lecos, Chris W. 1987. "Pretty Poison: Lead and Ceramic Ware." *BNET Business Network*. http://findarticles.com/p/articles/mi_m1370/is_v21/ai_5117848/pg_3.

Sheets, R. W. 1997. "Extraction of Lead, Cadmium, and Zinc from Overglaze Decorations on Ceramic Dinnerware by Acidic and Basic Food Substances." *Science of the Total Environment* 197 (1–3):167–175.

———.1999. "Acid Extraction of Lead and Cadmium from Newly-Purchased Ceramic and Melamine Dinnerware." *Science of the Total Environment* 234 (103):233–237.

Society of Glass and Ceramic Decorators. 2004. "Lead and Other Heavy Metals: Where Does the Decorating Industry Stand." *Guide to Heavy Metal Limits*. http://www.marckassoc.com/Documents/HeavyMetalLimits.doc.

ADHD by Any Other Name

Hull, Janet Starr. 1998. *Sweet Poison: How the World's Most Popular Artificial Sweetener Is Killing Us—My Story*. Far Hills, NJ: New Horizon Press.

———. 2005. *Splenda: Is It Safe or Not?* McKinney, TX: The Pickle Press.

SECTION III
HIDDEN TRIGGERS

Vaccinations: A Parent's Right to Choose

Association of American Physicians and Surgeons, Inc. 2008. "Poling Case Intensifies Debate; Vaccine-Autism Link Worth Investigating, Says Former NIH Director." *AAPS Online*. http://www.aapsonline.org/newsoftheday/0027.

Attkisson, Sharyl. 2008. "Leading Dr.: Vaccines-Autism Worth Study CBS News Exclusive: Former Head of NIH Says Government Too Quick to Dismiss Possible Link." *CBS News*. http://www.cbsnews.com.

Burton, Dan. 2000. "FACA: Conflicts of Interest and Vaccine Development: Preserving the Integrity of the Process." *U.S. House of Representatives Committee on Government Reform, June 15*.

———. 2005. "Wellness Information: Autism and Vaccines." *U.S. House of Representatives*. http://www.house.gov/burton/autism.htm.

Generation Rescue. "Cal-Oregon Vaccinated vs. Unvaccinated Survey." *Generation Rescue*. http://generationrescue.org/survey.html.

Grabenstein, J. D. 2006. "Vaccine Excipient and Media Summary." *Centers for Disease Control and Prevention*. http://www.cdc.gov/vaccines/pubs/pinkbook/downloads/appendices/B/excipient-table-1.pdf.

———. 2008. "Vaccine Excipient and Media Summary, Part 2." *Centers for Disease Control and Prevention*. http://www.cdc.gov/vaccines/pubs/pinkbook/downloads/appendices/B/excipient-table-2.pdf.

Incao, Philip. 2006. "How Vaccinations Work." *CompWellness.net*. http://www.comp wellness. net/mp/How%20Vaccinations%20Work.pdf.

Johns Hopkins Bloomberg School of Public Health. 2008. "Thimerosal Content in Some U.S. Licensed Vaccines." *Institute for Vaccine Safety*. http://www.vaccinesafety.edu/thi-table.htm.

Moskowitz, Richard. 1983. "The Case against Immunizations." *Journal of the AIH* (March).

National Vaccine Information Center. 2000. "Special Report: Autism and Vaccines: A New Look at an Old Story, The Vaccine Reaction." http://www.nvic.org.

Neustaedter, Randall. 2002. *The Vaccine Guide: Risks and Benefits for Children and Adults*. Berkeley, CA: North Atlantic Books.

Palevsky, Lawrence B. 2008. "Aluminum and Vaccine Ingredients: What Do We Know? What Don't We Know?" *National Vaccine Information Center*. http://www.nvic.org.

Sears, Robert W. 2008. "Is Aluminum the New Thimerosal?" *Mothering*. 146 (January – February):46–53.

Autism: The Misdiagnosis of Our Future Generations

Buttar, Rashid A. 2004. "Autism Spectrum Disorders: An Update of Federal Government Initiatives and Revolutionary New Treatments of Neurodevelopmental Diseases." *U.S. Congressional Sub-Committee Hearing, May 6*. www.drbuttar.com.

Fisher, Barbara Loe. 2008. "Vaccine Safety Research Priorities: Engaging the Public." *National Vaccine Information Center*. http://www.nvic.org.

Gluten and Dairy: Hidden Toxins and How They Contribute to Digestive Disorders

Braly, James, and Ron Hoggan. 2002. *Dangerous Grains*. New York: Penguin Group.

Haas, Elson, and Buck Levin. 2006. *Staying Healthy with Nutrition*. Berkeley, CA: Celestial Arts.

Jones, David S., Mark Hyman, and Sidney MacDonald Baker. 2005. "Functional Medicine and Biochemical Individuality: A Paradigm Shift." In *Textbook of Functional Medicine*. Gig Harbor, WA: The Institute for Functional Medicine.

Kristal, Harold, and James M. Haig. 2002. *The Nutrition Solution*. Berkeley, CA: North Atlantic Books.

Krohn, Jacqueline, Frances Taylor, and Erla Mae Larson. 1996. *Allergy Relief and Prevention*. Point Roberts, WA: Hartley and Marks Publishers.

Lombard, Jay, and Carl Germano. 1997. *The Brain Wellness Plan*. New York: Kensington Publishing Corp.

SECTION IV
BALANCING THE BRAIN AND BODY
Understanding Amino Acid Therapy

Amminge, G. P., G. E. Berger, and M. R. Schäfer. 2007. "Omega-3 Fatty Acids Supplementation in Children with Autism: A Double-Blind Randomized, Placebo Controlled Pilot Study." *Biol Psychiatry* 61 (4):551–553.

Delahanty, D., N. Nugent, N. Christopher, and M. Waltsh. 2005. "Initial Urinary Epinephrine and Cortisol Levels Predict Acute PTSD Symptoms in Child Trauma Victims." *Psychoneuroendocrinology* 121:2.

Oades, R. D. 2005. "The Control of Responsiveness in ADHD by Catecholamines: Evidence for Dopaminergic, Noradrenergic, and Interactive Roles." *Developmental Science* 8 (2):122–131.

Purvis, K. B., D. R. Cross, and G. Kellerman. 2006. "An Experimental Evaluation of Targeted Amino Acid Therapy with At-Risk Children. *Journal of Alternative and Complementary Medicine* 12 (6):591–592.

Purvis, K. B., D. R. Cross, and W. D. Sunshine. 2007. *The Connected Child*. New York: McGraw Hill.

Sinn, Natalie, and Janet Bryan. 2007. "Effect of Supplementation with Polyunsaturated Fatty Acids and Micronutrients on Learning and Behavior Problems Associated with Child ADHD." *Journal of Developmental and Behavioral Pediatrics* 28 (2):82–91.

United Business Media. "2008 Children's Nutrition Survey Reveals Majority of U.S. Parents Unaware of DHA Benefits to Children's Health." *PR Newswire*. http://sev.prnewswire .com/retail/20080421/LAM009A21042008-1.html.

Weidman-Becker, A. "Child Abuse and Neglect: Effects on Child Development, Brain Development, and Interpersonal Relationships." *International Adoption Article Directory*. http://www.adoptionarticlesdirectory.com/Article/Child-Abuse-and-Neglect—Effects-on-child-development—brain-development—and-interpersonal-relationships/42 (Accessed October 17, 2007).

ADHD and the Thyroid Gland

Cohen, Mark. 2007. "Misdiagnosing ADHD." *Discover Magazine*, Aug. 22.

Donovan, Jennifer. 1997. "Hyperactivity Linked to Thyroid Hormones." *Science Daily*, March 12.

Hauser, P., A. J. Zametkin, P. Martinez, B. Vitiello, J. A. Matochik, A. J. Mixson, and B. D. Weintraub. 1993. "Attention Deficit-Hyperactivity Disorder in People with Generalized Resistance to Thyroid Hormone." *New England Journal of Medicine* 328 (14):997–1001.

Hauser, P., R. Soler, F. Brucker-Davis, and B. D. Weintraub. 1997. "Thyroid Hormones Correlate with Symptoms of Hyperactivity But Not Inattention in Attention Deficit Hyperactivity Disorder." *Psychoneuroendocrinology* 22 (2):107–14.

Weiss, R. E., M. A. Stein, B. Trommer, and S. Refetoff. 1993. "Attention-Deficit Hyperactivity Disorder and Thyroid Function." *Junior Pediatrics* 123 (4):539–45.

Brain Seizures and the ADHD Connection

Cabeza, R., and A. Kingstone. 2001. *Handbook of Functional Neuroimaging*. Cambridge, MA: MIT Press.

Dunn, D. W., J. K. Austin, J. Harezlak, and W. T. Ambrosius. 2003. "ADHD and Epilepsy in Childhood." *Developmental Medicine and Child Neurology* 45:50–54.

Niedermeyer, N., and F. Lopes da Silva. 1987. *Electroencephalography: Basic Principles, Clinical Applications, and Related Fields*. Baltimore, MD: Lippincott, Williams and Wilkins.

Sterman, M. B. 1976. "Effects of Brain Surgery and EEG Operant Conditioning on Seizure Latency Following Monomethylhydrazine Intoxication in the Cat." *Experimental Neurology* 50:757–765.

————.2000. "Basic Concepts and Clinical Findings in the Treatment of Seizure Disorders with EEG Operant Conditioning." *Clinical Electroencephalography* 31 (1):45–55.

Electromagnetic Field Disturbances

Chan, Lisa. 2008. "Study Shows Risk of Cell Phone Use While Pregnant." *CBS News*. http://cbs5.com/technology/pregnant.cell.phone.2.727935.html.

Foggo, Daniel. 2007. "Cancer Clusters at Phone Masts." *Times Online*. http://technology.timesonline.co.uk/tol/news/tech_and_web/personal_tech/article1687491.ece.

Fox News. 2008. "Cell Phones Could Be More Dangerous than Cigarettes," *FoxNews.com*. http://www.foxnews.com/story/0,2933,343335,00.html.

Franch, Peter. "Cells Are Permanently Damaged by Cell Phone Frequencies," *CPR News Bureau*. http://www.cprnews.com.

Kovach, Sue. 2007. "The Hidden Dangers of Cell Phone Radiation." *LEF Magazine*, August.

Worthington, Amy. 2007. "Radiation Poisoning of America." *Global Research*. http://global research.ca/index.php?context=va&aid=7025.

SECTION V
ALTERNATIVE APPROACHES TO HEALING

ADHD: Spurious Diagnosis, Specious Treatment

Almli, C. R. 1990. "Normal Sequential Behavioral and Physiological Changes throughout the Developmental Arc." *Neurological Rehabilitation, 2nd ed*. Ed. Darcy Ann Umphred. St. Louis, MO: C.V. Mosby.

Ayres, A. Jean. 1973. *Sensory Integration and Learning Disorders*. Los Angeles: Western Psychological Press.

Bertherat, Therese, and Carol Bernstein. 1989. *The Body Has Its Reasons*. Rochester, VT: Healing Arts Press.

Berthoz, A. 2000. *The Brain's Sense of Movement, Perspectives in Cognitive Neuroscience*. Cambridge, MA: Harvard University Press.

Bluestone, Judith. 2004. *The Fabric of Autism: Weaving the Threads into a Cogent Theory*. Seattle, WA: Sapphire Enterprises.

Diller, Lawrence H. 1998. *Running on Ritalin: A Physician Reflects on Children, Society, and Performance in a Pill*. New York: Bantam Books.

Doidge, Norman. 2007. *The Brain that Changes Itself*. New York: Penguin Groups.

Kranowitz, Carol S. 1998. *The Out-of-Synch Child: Recognizing and Coping with Sensory Integration Dysfunction*. New York: Skylight Press.

LeDoux, Joseph. 2003. *The Synaptic Self: How Our Brain Becomes Who We Are*. New York: Penguin Group.

Lemer, P. S., ed. 2008. *Envisioning a Bright Future: Interventions that Work for Children and Adults with Autism Spectrum Disorders*. Santa Ana, CA: OEP Foundation, Inc.

Levinson, Harold N. 1990. *Total Concentration: How to Understand Attention Deficit Disorders*. New York: M. Evans and Co.

Lewis, D., J. P. Bluestone, M. Savina, W. H. Zoller, E. B. Meshberg, and S. Minoshima. 2006. "Imaging Cerebral Activity in Recovery from Chronic Traumatic Brain Injury: A Preliminary Report." *Journal of Neuroimaging* 16 (3):272–277.

Mate, Gabor. 1999. *Scattered Minds: A New Look at the Origins and Healing of Attention Deficit Disorder*. Toronto: Alfred A. Knopf.

Randolph, Shirley L., and Margot C. Heineger. 1994. *Kids Learn from the Inside Out: How to Enhance the Human Matrix*. Boise, ID: Legendary Publishing.

Stevens, Laura J. 2000. *Twelve Effective Ways to Help Your ADD/ADHD Child: Drug-Free Alternatives for Attention-Deficit Disorders*. New York: Penguin Group.

Stitt, Barbara R. 1997. *Food and Behavior: A Natural Connection*. Manitowoc, WI: Natural Press.

Walker, S. 1998. *The Hyperactivity Hoax*. New York: St. Martin's Press.

The Brain Gym Method

Dennison, Paul E. and Gail E. Dennison. *1989. Brain Gym Teacher's Edition*. Ventura, CA: Edu-Kinesthetics, Inc.

———.2007. *Brain Gym 101 Balance for Daily Life Manual*. Ventura, CA: Edu-Kinesthetics, Inc.

Dennison, Paul E. 2006. *Brain Gym and Me.* Ventura, CA: Edu-Kinesthetics, Inc.

Hannaford, Carla. 1995. *Smart Moves Why Learning Is Not All in Your Head.* Arlington, VA: Great Ocean Publishers, Inc.

Koster, Cecilia Freeman. 2004. *Interfacing Brain Gym with Children Who Have Special Needs.* Ventura, CA: Edu-Kinesthetics, Inc.

Emotional Freedom Techniques: Healing the Underlying Emotional Contributors to ADD and ADHD

Ball, Ron, et al. 2006. *Freedom at Your Fingertips.* Fredericksburg, VA: Inroads Publishing.

Carlo, George, and Martin Schram. 2001. *Cell Phones: Invisible Hazards in the Wireless Age.* New York: Carroll and Graf.

Church, Dawson. 2007. *The Genie in Your Genes.* Santa Rosa, CA: Elite Books.

Eden, Donna, and David Feinstein. 1998. *Energy Medicine.* New York: Penguin Putnam.

Feinstein, David, Donna Eden, and Gary Craig. 2005. *The Promise of Energy Psychology: Revolutionary Tools for Dramatic Personal Change.* New York: Penguin Group.

Fisher, Howard. 2007. *The Invisible Threat: The Risks Associated with EMFs.* Toronto: Wood Publishing.

Goldberg, Gerald, MD. 2006. *Would You Put Your Head in a Microwave Oven?* Bloomington, IN: Author-House.

SECTION VI
MORE ALTERNATIVE APPROACHES TO HEALING
Homeopathy and ADHD

Collier, Bob. "ADHD Statistics." *ADHD-Report.com.* http://www.adhd-report.com/adhd/ 1_adhd_statistics.html.

Gerber, Richard. 2001. *Vibrational Medicine, The #1 Handbook of Subtle Energy Therapies.* Rochester, VT: Bear and Co.

Ullman, Dana. 1995. *The Consumer's Guide to Homeopathy.* New York: Putnam and Sons.

Adverse Reactions to Ritalin and Other Medications

Breggin, Peter R., MD. 2001. *Talking Back to Ritalin.* Cambridge, MA: Da Capo Press.

CNN News. 2008. "Heart Screening Urged before Kids Get ADHD Drugs." *CNN.com.* www.cnn.com/2008/HEALTH/conditions/04/21/adhd.drugs.heart.ap/index.html.

Eli Lilly and Company. 2008. "Important Safety Information on Strattera for Children Ages 6 and Older, Adolescents, and Adults." *Strattera.com.* www.strattera.com/hcp/strattera_ safety_information.jsp.

MediLexicon International Ltd. 2006. "ADHD Drugs Should Have Black Box Warning, Says FDA Advisory Panel." *Medical News TODAY.* www.medicalnewstoday.com/ articles/37584.php.

National Alliance against Mandated Mental Health Screening and Psychiatric Drugging of Children. *Death from Ritalin: The Truth behind ADHD.* www.Ritalindeath.com.

WordPress.com. 2008. "Link between Prozac, Ritalin, Luvox, Zoloft, and Paxil to School Shootings." *HealthWatcher.net*. http://healthwatcher.wordpress.com/2008/02/15/link-between-prozac-ritalin-luvox-zoloft-and-paxil-to-school-shootings.

The Intention Protocol

Backster, Cleve. 2003. *Primary Perception*. Anza, CA: White Rose Millennium Press.

Greene, Brian. 1999. *The Elegant Universe*. New York: W.W. Norton and Co.

McTaggart, Lynne. 2002. *The Field*. New York: HarperCollins Publishers.

———. 2007. *The Intention Experiment*. New York: Simon and Schuster.

Radin, Dean.1997. *The Conscious Universe*. New York: HarperCollins Publishers.

Walker, Evan Harris. 2000. *The Physics of Consciousness*. New York: Perseus Books.

Wolf, Fred Alan. 1981. *Taking the Quantum Leap*. New York: Harper and Row.

About the Contributors

Deborah Merlin

For fifteen years, Deborah Merlin made it her mission to be an advocate for her twins' special needs. As a new mother of very premature twins with challenging health problems, she found that doctors and other professionals offered only drugs as the solution. To find alternative ways to heal her children, she attended alternative medicine and nutritional seminars, performed extensive research on ADHD and other health-related issues, and kept impeccable records.

In 1993, she was the co-chair of the Westside Cities Council to help promote Public Law 99457, part H, which implemented early intervention services from birth through three years of age for children at risk. She co-ran a parent support group at the Westside Regional Center in Culver City, California, that focused on children with special needs and those at risk.

In 1990 and 1991, she was the coordinator for outreach to pediatricians (under Public Law 99457, part H) and coordinated presentations at hospitals to educate pediatricians on early intervention services and resources for children at risk from infancy to three years of age. She was a guest speaker on radio programs to promote early intervention.

Deborah was employed by Equifax Services as an insurance investigator from 1977 to 1991, which helped develop her research and analytical skills. She is a frequent guest speaker on radio shows throughout the United States and Canada. Deborah is also a consultant to parents who need support and provides resources regarding their children's individual needs. She is also an artist.

Judith Bluestone

Judith Bluestone was an educator, therapist, lecturer, author, and consultant. She had over forty years of experience in working with children and adults with neurodevelopmental challenges, in addition to her own extraordinary childhood, replete with sensory disturbances and bizarre behaviors that in the late twentieth century would have been labeled as autism, ADHD, obsessive-compulsive disorder, and others. Her academic studies and collaborative work in the fields of education, neurodevelopment, psychology, and rehabilitation methodologies led a Washington State county hospital to deem her a neurodevelopmental/educational therapist.

After resolving her own serious neurodevelopmental differences, and realizing she was not alone in facing such challenges, Judith developed the Holistic Approach to NeuroDevelopment and Learning Efficiency (HANDLE). Refusing to accept rejection of herself (although she was often socially ostracized) or of her ideas, in 1994 Judith founded The HANDLE Institute in Seattle and began to train others in her paradigm for understanding human functionality and building stable neurodevelopmental foundations for learning.

In 2004, Judith won regional and national Jefferson Awards and the Jacqueline Kennedy Onassis Award for creating and sharing HANDLE with her community, her country, and the world. There are now approximately 140 certified providers of HANDLE on five continents—and more in training. To accommodate this growth, Judith established The HANDLE Institute International, LLC, also in 2004.

HANDLE invites you to help extraordinary people do ordinary things, naturally.

Contact information: The HANDLE Institute
1300 Dexter Avenue N
110 The Casey Family Building
Seattle, WA 98109
206-204-6000
http://www.handle.org

James P. Blumenthal, DC, CCN, DACBN, FABFN

James P. Blumenthal received his bachelor's degree from Washington University in St. Louis, his doctor of chiropractic degree from Logan College, and his post-doctoral neurology training from Carrick Institute. He is a board certified clinical nutritionist, a diplomate of the American Clinical Board of Nutrition, a member of the American Chiropractic College of Nutrition, and a fellow of the American Board of Functional Neurology. He was named a research associate in biological medicine by Occidental Institute Research Foundation and served on the board of directors of the International College of Applied Kinesiology. He collaborates with an international team to advance teaching and research on retained primitive reflexes and applies Defeat Autism Now! principles to his work.

A third generation healer, Dr Blumenthal has studied and practiced as an herbalist, emergency medical technician, body-worker, doctor of chiropractic, clinical nutritionist, and functional neurologist. He has training in Chinese medicine and naturopathy and has served on the faculty of chiropractic, naturopathic, and Chinese medical schools.

Dr. Blumenthal specializes in treating children and adults with complex "syndrome disorders" (e.g., AD(H)D, Autism, Asperger's); digestive, immune, detoxification, and endocrine problems; and neurologic challenges (learning; memory, focus and attention; planning and sequencing; balance, vertigo, coordination; brain injuries). His high success rate can be attributed to listening carefully to his patients, treating each one as an individual and a partner in their healing process, and to the variety of healing traditions that he has been trained in.

Dr. Blumenthal uses extensive laboratory testing to guide his drug-free therapies. All of the tests and tools described in this book are available through his office. Having provided technical support to labs conducting amino acid, neurotransmitter, and hormone assays, he knows which tests will give the most useful information about a particular patient with the least invasiveness and the lowest cost.

Contact information: Brain Performance Center
Applied Kinesiology Center of Los Angeles
2990 S. Sepulveda Blvd., Suite 203
Los Angeles, CA, 90064
(310) 445-3350
DrBlu427@aol.com
http://www.AKCSM.com

Rashid Buttar, DO, FAAPM, FACAM, FAAIM

Rashid A. Buttar received his undergraduate degree from Washington University in St. Louis with a double major in biology and theology, and then attended medical school at the University of Osteopathic Medicine and Health Sciences, College of Osteopathic Medicine and Surgery, in Des Moines, Iowa. He trained in general surgery and emergency medicine and served as Brigade Surgeon for the 2nd Infantry Division, Republic of South Korea, and later as the Chief of the Department of Emergency Medicine at Moncrief Army Community Hospital at Ft. Jackson in Columbia, South Carolina. During his military career, Dr. Buttar had the privilege of serving with and being attached to the 2nd Infantry Division, the 101st Air Assault Division, and the 5th Special Forces Group.

Dr. Buttar is board certified and a diplomate in preventive medicine and clinical metal toxicology, is board eligible in emergency medicine, and has achieved fellowship status in three separate medical organizations: Fellow of the American College for Advancement in Medicine, Fellow of the American Academy of Preventive Medicine, and Fellow of the American Association of Integrative Medicine. Dr. Buttar practices in Charlotte, North Carolina, where he is the medical director of Advanced Concepts in Medicine, a clinic specializing in the treatment of cancer, heart disease, and other chronic conditions in patients refractory to conventional treatments, with a special emphasis on the interrelationship between metal toxicity and insidious disease processes. He also serves as Director of Clinical Research and Development for V-SAB Medical Laboratories, where he's extensively involved in research with polypeptide sequencing and identification technologies as well as innovative methodologies for drug delivery mechanisms. In addition, Dr. Buttar is involved in clinical research and outcome-based studies with various groups, including private bio-tech companies, university-based projects, and government-sponsored clinical research.

Dr. Buttar lectures worldwide on these subjects at scientific congresses and professional symposiums and is a frequently invited presenter at medical conferences. He has appeared and been featured in local, national, and international media including newspapers, radio, and television. Dr. Buttar has been invited to and testified in front of the North Carolina Congress as well as the United States

Congress, giving special testimony before the Congressional Sub-committee on Human Rights and Wellness. Phillips Publishing and Stephen Sinatra, MD, have listed Dr. Buttar as being among the top fifty doctors in the United States.

Dr. Buttar has been in charge of the national training program that leads to board certification in clinical metal toxicology through the American Board of Clinical Metal Toxicology and is also a member of the twelve-member National Metals Task Force, appointed to address the endemic nature of metal toxicity and the resulting implications on world health. Dr. Buttar currently serves as the chairman of the American Board of Clinical Metal Toxicology and is the president of the North Carolina Integrative Medical Society. He sits on numerous boards and CME committees for several medical organizations and societies, including the American Association for Health Freedom.

Dr. Buttar continues to actively teach as faculty for mainstream medical courses, such as Advanced Trauma Life Support (ATLS) for physicians through the American College of Surgeons, as well as teaching pediatric advanced life support and advanced cardiac life support courses to other physicians, nurses, and emergency response personnel. Dr. Buttar's DVD *Autism, The Misdiagnosis of Our Future Generations* is available at www. TheMedicalSeries.com.

Contact information: Center for Advanced Medicine and Clinical Research
20721 Torrence Chapel Road, Suite # 101–103
Cornelius, NC 28031
704-895-9355 (clinic phone)
www.drbuttar.com

Pat Farrell

For over twelve years, Pat Farrell has been an advocate of and coach for health-supporting lifestyles, primarily focusing on the emotional aspects to achieve health and well-being. Building upon conventional therapeutic methods, Pat utilizes techniques from Emotional Freedom Techniques, energy medicine, applied kinesiology, clinical hypnotherapy, and BioPro technology to help people achieve happiness and health.

Pat Farrell presented her unique solution to stress to companies such as Harley Davidson, The Newspaper Association of America/NIE, Kaiser Permanente, Sharp Health Care, Cary Medical Center, Blue Cross, and the U.S. Department of the Interior. The change in people is often immediate and usually permanent. Many refer to Pat's process as "the miracle drug. . . *without the drug.*"

Pat is the author of the internationally acclaimed book *101 Ways to Get a Life: How to Be Happy . . . No Matter What's Happening* and is a popular guest on radio and television.

Contact information: 760-961-4027 or 877-2-B-HAPPY
www.pat-farrell.com
www.mybiopro.com/patfarrell

Stuart H. Garber, DC, PhD

Stuart Garber has been practicing holistic medicine since 1981. He has lectured to medical, dental, chiropractic, and acupuncture groups in the United States, Europe, Asia, and the Caribbean.

In 1997, Dr. Garber became the first person in the United States to receive a doctorate degree in homeopathy. He is the developer of Dr. Garber's Natural Solutions, a line of condition-specific biotherapy formulas. Dr. Garber practices in Santa Monica, California, where he also conducts research in homeopathic medicine.

Contact information: 517 Ocean Front Walk, Suite 11
Venice, CA 90291
310-396-7247
info@drgarber.net

Dan O. Harper, MD, PhD

Dan Harper was born and raised in East Texas. He acquired polio in the epidemic of 1952 and had five years of learning how to walk again. His 107-degree fever caused or allowed certain learning disorders to appear as dyslexia and ADD; his mother called it "Dennis the Menace" syndrome. He graduated from Abilene Christian College magna cum laude and from Baylor College of Medicine cum laude. Dr. Harper served a residency in family practice at the University of Oregon Health Sciences Center in Portland. After a period of time in Nigeria at the Nigerian Christian Hospital in Onichingwa, Dr. Harper returned to do emergency room work and family practice.

Dr. Harper is board certified in family medicine and holistic medicine and has a doctorate in homeopathy. He has accumulated over thirty-five thousand hours of ER experience and over thirty-five hundred hours of continuing medical education in the last five years, mostly in complementary medicine.

Currently, Dr. Harper does only holistic practice, spending one to two hours on the initial consultation. He prescribes lifestyle adjustments, dietary changes, and nutritional supplements to allow the body to return to its natural healing mode.

Contact information: 511 South Cedros Suite B
Solana Beach, CA 92075
858-755-1126
www.drdanharper.com
www.drdanharper.meta-ehealth.com

Janet Starr Hull, PhD

Janet Starr Hull has a very diverse background with academic degrees and experience in geology, international geography, environmental science, fitness training, and nutrition. She is an OSHA-certified environmental hazardous waste emergency response specialist and toxicologist, a former firefighter, and a college professor.

In 1991, Dr. Hull had an unexpected change in career after she was diagnosed with "incurable" Graves' disease. Through diligent research and her thorough understanding of toxicity, she later discovered that her "Graves' disease" was actually aspartame poisoning. She has since worked to inform consumers about the health dangers of artificial sweeteners.

Dr. Hull's experiences have provided pieces to a life-long puzzle—the damaging effects of artificial sweeteners. She combined her various skills to form a unique application to natural medicine. Her work is based upon the interrelationships of all sciences, as she personally discovered "what works in nature can surely work in man."

Contact information: www.janethull.com
                                www.healthynewsletter.com

Jack Johnstone, PhD

Jack Johnstone received his bachelor's degree in biology and psychology at Antioch College and his doctorate in psychology at the University of California at San Francisco. He is currently the president and CEO of Q-Metrx, Inc., and is an associate researcher in the Department of Psychology at UCLA. Dr. Johnstone is a consultant to Aspect Medical Systems, Inc. and California Clinical Trials.

Contact information: Q-METRX
                                1612 W. Olive Street, Suite 301
                                Burbank, CA 91506
                                818-563-5409
                                www.q-metrx.com

Kathleen Lewis, DC, CBT

Kathleen Lewis teaches classes in The Intention Protocol, meditation, and quantum consciousness, including how to access the quantum field using techniques that combine the mind and the heart. You may hear her radio show, Spinning Light, archived on her website. Dr. Lewis is a chiropractor certified in First Line Therapy and Matrix Energetics. She is also a Quantum Biofeedback Specialist. Dr. Lewis has a practice in Los Angeles, California.

Contact information: 12114 Venice Blvd.
                                Los Angeles, CA 90066
                                310-391-1452
                                www.spinninglight.com

Debbie Lindgren, ClHom

Debbie Lindgren became interested in complementary healing strategies after one of her sons was diagnosed with lead poisoning. Debbie is a married mother of two, a homeopath, and cofounder of Bluedominoes, Inc., a company that creates lead-free children's art supplies and provides evidence-based information to promote healthier solutions for a higher level of safety, quality, and peace of mind.

The Bluedominoes philosophy is that environmental and dietary factors influence children's health, learning, and behavior. By connecting these links, Bluedominoes provides actionable strategies for parents.

Contact information: www.bluedominoes.com

Marlene McKee, Certified Nutrition Educator, DIHom

Marlene McKee was raised and educated in Germany. After college, she studied in England at the British Institute of Homeopathy at Staines, and received a diploma in the advanced course of studies in homeopathic medicine. When Marlene came to the United States for a visit, she loved it and eventually decided to stay. She continued her education in biological sciences and nutrition at the Institute of Educational Therapy, Bauman College, Penngrove, California, where she became a certified nutrition educator.

Marlene has owned and operated health food stores in Ann Arbor, Michigan, and Los Angeles. Her mother passed on to her a vast knowledge of medicinal herbs and natural healing. She showed her how to use herbs and food as prevention and cures. Her family never had to see a doctor, nor did they take Western medicines or antibiotics. Marlene's mother told her about vitamins in foods before anybody else ever talked about them. Because of her upbringing, she knew that people could heal themselves with the proper food, nature's medicines, and the body's innate wisdom.

Marlene has been in the business of educating people in health-promoting eating and natural remedies for twenty-seven years.

Contact information: 310-577-0852
www.bodyiqonline.com

Trisha Ochoa, CHN

Trisha Ochoa is a board-certified holistic nutritionist and, as a registered member of the National Association of Nutrition Professionals, she continues her training by working closely with other professionals in her field. She earned her bachelor's degree from the University of California at Berkeley and her nutrition certification from the American Academy of Nutrition.

She specializes in holistic nutrition, emphasizing the need for optimum nutrition to ensure optimum health, not just the absence of illness. By recognizing the mechanisms by which the individual systems of the body work together, she designs eating patterns and supplementation methods to bring total health to her clients. Trisha practices nutrition counseling and lectures in Santa Monica, California.

Contact information: 310-428-9098
Santa Monica, California
trishaochoacnc@yahoo.com

Emily Roberts, MA, LPC-I

Emily Roberts received her undergraduate degree in psychology and her master's degree in counseling from St. Edwards University in Austin, Texas. Emily has worked with Pam Machemehl-Helmly, CN and chief science officer at Neurogistics, for three years; she is also a certified Neurogistics practitioner.

Emily is dedicated to helping children in need and providing families with support. Her background in counseling psychology allows her to incorporate the science of neurotransmitter testing into her practice while also assisting parents and families through the Balance Your Child's Brain program. As a Neurogistics practitioner, Emily is able to assist parents all across the country and provide brain-chemistry balancing and education to any child in need of services. Her passion is working with children from troubled backgrounds, including adopted and foster children.

Contact information: Neurogistics Corporation
888-257-9068
http://www.balanceyourchildsbrain.com
http://www.neurogistics.com

Barbara Schwartz, MA

Barbara Schwartz is the founder of Equilibrium. She is a pioneer in the education and development of effective, non-medication, integrative brain-body techniques for overcoming symptoms of autism, ADD/ADHD, and other physical, emotional, learning, and/or behavioral conditions that affect both children and adults in alarming numbers.

Barbara has over twenty years of credentialed classroom teaching experience and is an educational kinesiologist, developmental specialist, a certified Brain Gym instructor, scotopic sensitivity syndrome evaluator, essential oil consultant, and holistic health practitioner.

Equilibrium can provide safe, proven, drug-free solutions to individuals, families, and groups. Barbara has created classroom, home study, daycare, and camp programs for children, parent workshops, and teacher training, as well as adult workshops. Barbara Schwartz is an author, frequent lecturer, and television personality. She also works directly with adults, children, and families on a private consultation basis. Barbara's belief can be summed up as follows: When your brain and body are in balance, your life is in Equilibrium.

Contact information: 818-345-0743
www.EquilibriumHealing.com

Jane Sheppard

Jane Sheppard is the editor and publisher of Healthy Child, a comprehensive website, newsletter, and blog for parents about natural, holistic health for children. Healthy Child helps to empower parents to make informed choices to protect the health and well-being of their children. Healthy Child offers parents thoroughly researched, safe, nontoxic products for babies and children.

Jane is the author of *Super Healthy Kids: Strengthening Your Child's Resistance to Disease, Protect Your Baby from Toxic Exposures,* and numerous parenting articles. Jane lives in Northern California.

Contact information: www.HealthyChild.com
Santa Rosa, CA
707-570-0408

Lesa Werner, ND

Lesa Werner is a licensed, board-certified doctor of naturopathic medicine. She maintains licenses to practice naturopathic medicine in both California and Connecticut, along with an additional license for dispensing approved pharmaceuticals in California.

Dr. Werner is a graduate of Bastyr University in Seattle, where she earned her doctoral degree in naturopathic medicine. Bastyr University has the distinction of being the leading educational and research institution for science-based natural medicine.

Dr. Werner received her baccalaureate degree in biology from Western Connecticut State University and an associate degree in ophthalmic design and dispensing from Middlesex College in Connecticut. After a varied work history that included employment as an optician, a certified ophthalmic technician, and an EMT in Connecticut and New York, she ultimately found her calling in the field of natural medicine.

Following graduation from Bastyr, Dr. Werner established a successful practice in Connecticut before moving to California. While in Connecticut, she functioned as a primary care physician, focusing on the treatment of allergies, ADD/ADHD, autism, menopause and hormone balancing, Lyme disease, fibromyalgia, high cholesterol, pediatric illnesses, and digestive disorders. In California, Dr. Werner's practice primarily encompasses women's health care and pediatric illnesses.

Contact information: 8961 Sunset Boulevard, Suite 2E
West Hollywood, CA 90069
310-801-9514
www.drlesawerner.com

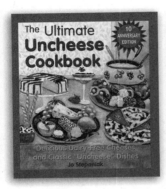
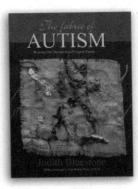
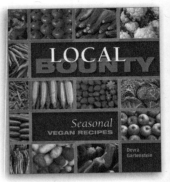
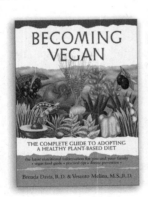
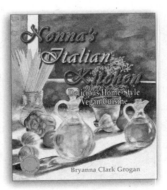
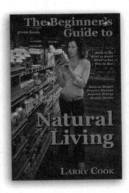